The Management of Headache

GW00382253

Editor

F. Clifford Rose, FRCP

Director
Princess Margaret Migraine Clinic
Department of Neurology
Charing Cross Hospital
London, England

New York 🕮 Raven Press

Raven Press, 1185 Avenue of the Americas, New York, New York 10036

Made in the United States of America

Library of Congress Cataloging-in-Publication Data

The management of headache.

Includes bibliographies and index.
1. Migraine. 2. Headache. 3. Cluster headache.
I. Rose, F. Clifford (Frank Clifford) [DNLM: 1. Headache.
WL 342 M266]
RC392.M28 1988 616.07´2 86-42503
ISBN 0-88167-246-7
ISBN 0-88167-385-4 (soft)

9 8 7 6 5 4 3 2 1

THE MANAGEMENT OF HEADACHE

Preface

Headache is probably the most common of all symptoms, and we are pleased to present in this volume the most current findings which represent the considerable increase in the knowledge of its pathogenesis and management. It is our hope that patients who suffer from headache will benefit from the widespread circulation of this knowledge. This volume will be of great use to family practitioners and general physicians.

After discussions on classification (Chapter 1), physical findings (Chapter 2) and differential diagnosis (Chapter 3), the following three chapters show how recent advances have changed our views on the pathogenesis of migraine. Previously the aura was considered to be due to intracerebral vasoconstriction and the headache due to extracranial vasodilatation. The work of the Danish School (see Chapter 5) has thrown doubt on this and there are now other possibilities to be considered, e.g., the spreading depression of Leão (see Chapters 5 and 6). The complications (Chapter 7) and therapy (Chapters 8–10) of migraine are fully considered. Separate chapters on cluster headache (Chapter 11) and muscle contraction headache (Chapter 12) are followed by consideration of headache in the Emergency Department (Chapter 13).

It is now recognized that headaches in children are not uncommon, and this subject is reviewed in depth (see Chapter 14). The study of headache is no longer a Cinderella of neurological research and its future is assured (see Chapter 15).

F. Clifford Rose

Acknowledgments

This book is based on a series of lectures given following the biennial International Symposium organized by the Migraine Trust in September of 1984 at the Charing Cross Hospital and Westminister Medical School. We are particularly grateful to the British Migraine Association and Sandoz (U.K.) for their support.

Contents

Contributors

Michael Anthony, OBE, MD, FRCP, FRACP, *Associate Professor, Department of Neurology, The Prince Henry Hospital, and the School of Medicine, University of New South Wales, Sydney, N.S.W. 2036 Australia*

Otto Appenzeller, MD, PhD, *Professor of Neurology and Medicine, University of New Mexico School of Medicine, Albuquerque, New Mexico 87131*

George W. Bruyn, MD, DSc, *Chairman, Department of Neurology, Academic Hospital, State University, AA 2333 Leiden, The Netherlands*

J. Keith Campbell, MD, FRCP (Edin), *Department of Neurology, Mayo Clinic, 200 First Street, S. W., Rochester, Minnesota 55905*

J. D. Carroll, MD, FRCP, FRCPE, FRCPI, *Royal Surrey County Hospital, Farnham Road, Guildford, Surrey, England*

Michael Chopp, MD, *Department of Neurology, Henry Ford Hospital, 2799 West Grand Boulevard, Detroit, Michigan 48202*

John Edmeads, MD, *Professor of Neurology, Sunnybrook Medical Center, University of Toronto, Ontario M4N 3M5, Canada*

James R. Ewing, MD, *Department of Neurology, Henry Ford Hospital, 2799 West Grand Boulevard, Detroit, Michigan 48202*

M. D. Ferrari, MD, *Department of Neurology, Academic Hospital, State University, Leiden, The Netherlands*

John Fozard, PhD, *Centre de Recherche, Merrell-Dow Research Institute, Strasbourg Research Center, 16 rue d'Ankara, 67084 Strasbourg-Cedex, France*

J. A. Gray, MA, MB, BS, MRCP (UK), *Research Registrar in Neurology, Regional Neurological Unit, and Associate Lecturer, University of Surrey, Guildford, Surrey, England*

J. A. Helpern, MD, *Department of Neurology, Henry Ford Hospital, 2799 West Grand Boulevard, Detroit, Michigan 48202*

Judith Hockaday, MD, FRCP, *Consultant in Paediatric Neurology, John Radcliffe Hospital, Oxford 0X3 9DU England*

James W. Lance, CBE, MD, FRCP, FRACP, FAA, *Chairman, Department of Neurology, The Prince Henry Hospital, and Professor of Neurology, University of New South Wales, Sydney, N.S.W. 2036 Australia*

Jes Olesen, MD, *Department of Neuromedicine, Københavns amts sygehus i Gentofte, 2900 Hellerup, Denmark*

R. Peatfield, MD, MRCP, *Department of Neurology, St. Jame's Hospital, Leeds LS9 7TF England*

F. Clifford Rose, FRCP, *Director, Princess Margaret Migraine Clinic, Department of Neurology, Charing Cross Hospital, London W6 8RF England*

K. M. A. Welch, MD, *Chairman, Department of Neurology, Henry Ford Hospital, 2799 West Grand Boulevard, Detroit, Michigan 48202*

Marcia Wilkinson, MA, DM, FRCP, *City of London Migraine Clinic, 22 Charterhouse Square, London EC1M 6DX England*

Dewey K. Ziegler, MD, *Chairman and Professor, Department of Neurology, University of Kansas College of Health Sciences and Hospital, 39th and Rainbow Boulevard, Kansas City, Kansas 66103*

K. J. Zilkha, M.D., FRCP, *King's College Hospital, Denmark Hill, London SE5 9RS England*

The Management of Headache, edited by F. Clifford Rose. Raven Press, New York © 1988.

NOSOLOGY OF HEADACHE

James W. Lance, CBE, MD, FRCP, FRACP, FAA

Chairman, Department of Neurology,
The Prince Henry Hospital, and
Professor of Neurology, University of New South Wales,
Sydney, Australia

Nosology means a systematic classification or arrangement of diseases. While descriptions of headaches are found in medical literature from 3,000 B.C. onwards, attempts to classify the causes of headache are quite recent. At the end of the last century, Gowers (29) separated headaches caused by cerebral tumor and other brain diseases from migraine and toxemic, congestive, gastric, neuralgic, anemic, and neurasthenic causes. He also mentioned brain-work and brain exhaustion, stating that, in some cases, the amount of brain work "has not been large, but is excessive on account of the nerve-strength of the individual".

Our present understanding of headache mechanisms is based to a large extent on the observations and research of Harold G. Wolff (74) who was a member of The Ad Hoc Committee on Classification of Headache, chaired by Arnold Friedman (27). The Ad Hoc Committee put forward a classification (Table 1) which started with migraine and related headaches and progressed to headaches caused by structural abnormalities.

TABLE 1.   Classification of Headache by the Ad Hoc Committee

I.		Vascular Headache of Migraine Type
	A.	"Classic" migraine
	B.	"Common" migraine
	C.	"Cluster" headache
	D.	"Hemiplegic" and "ophthalmoplegic" migraine
	E.	"Lower-half" headache
II.		Muscle-contraction headache
III.		Combined headache: Vascular and muscle-contraction
IV.		Headache of nasal vasomotor reaction
V.		Headache of delusional, conversion, or hypochondriacal states
VI.		Nonmigrainous vascular headaches
VII.		Traction headache
VIII.		Headache due to overt cranial inflammation
IX-XIII.		Headache due to disease of ocular, aural, nasal and sinus, dental, or other cranial or neck structures
XIV.		Cranial neuritides
XV.		Cranial neuralgias

1

Lance (41) tackled the problem in the reverse direction, beginning with headaches that are clearly explicable by organic disease of the nerves, vessels or surrounding tissues and ending with those of more dubious pathophysiology. This has the advantage of placing the known before the unknown, but means that the most common forms of headache are considered last. This approach will be used in the present Chapter and is summarized in Table 2.

TABLE 2.   Summary of Headache Classification Presented Here

Local cranial disorders
Disorders of extracranial vessels
Pain from the cranial nerves
    Excessive stimulation
    Compression
    Inflammation
    Idiopathic neuralgia
    Atypical facial pain
Referred pain
    Eyes
    Sinus, nasopharynx
    Teeth, temporo-mandibular joints
    Neck
Intracranial causes
    Vasodilatation
    Meningeal irritation
    Traction on, or displacement of, intracranial vessels
    Benign cough headache
Episodic 'vascular' headache
    Migraine
    Cluster headache
Tension headache
Psychogenic headache

Local Cranial Disorders

Expanding lesions within the cranial bones may stretch the periosteum and cause localized pain. Paget's disease may be associated with headache, probably as a result of increased blood flow to the affected area. Occasionally inflammation of the scalp or skull may be a source of pain and headache may also result from injury to the nerves or vessels of the scalp.

Disorders of Extracranial Vessels

Temporal (giant-cell) arteritis. This condition, of unknown etiology, is unusual before the age of 50 years. Pain and tenderness may be confined to affected arteries or may spread diffusely over the head. Aching of muscles and joints ("polymyalgia rheumatica") is associated in about half the patients (69).

Carotidynia. This term simply implies pain radiating upwards from the neck to the face, with tenderness over the carotid artery (59). It may be symptomatic of trauma to, or dissection of, the common carotid artery. In other instances it arises spontaneously and runs a self-limited course, possibly caused by a viral infection, or it may recur intermittently with throbbing headache in a manner suggesting a migraine variant (57). An elongated styloid process may give rise to pain in the cheek, chin or neck along the distribution of the carotid artery, known as Eagle's syndrome (48).

Pain from the Cranial Nerves

The dura, intracranial arteries and veins of the anterior and middle cranial fossa are supplied by the first division of the trigeminal nerve and may thus refer pain to the eye and forehead. Irritation of the glossopharyngeal nerve causes pain deep to the angle of the jaw, one side of the throat and base of the tongue. The vagus and nervus intermedius refer pain to the ear.

Excessive stimulation.
Peripheral branches of the trigeminal nerve may give rise to headache if the subject wears a band around the head or tight hat, or dives into cold water. Swallowing ice-cream or an ice-cold drink may cause pain known as ice-cream headache, more common in those susceptible to migraine (56). The headache is usually mid-frontal but is referred to the habitual site of headache in one-third of migrainous patients (20).

Compression.
The first division of the trigeminal nerve may be compressed in the orbit, the superior orbital fissure, cavernous sinus or at the apex of the petrous temporal bone. Expansion of an aneurysm of the internal carotid artery causes pain behind the eye. Slowly growing lesions such as meningioma may not give rise to headache until late in their course. Three eponymous syndromes should be mentioned:
Tolosa-Hunt syndrome. Recurrent painful ophthalmoplegia is named after the description given by Tolosa (65) and Hunt et al. (36). In most cases, the third, fourth and sixth cranial nerves are involved together with the first division of the trigeminal nerves, probably by a granuloma in the region of the superior orbital fissure (19).
Raeder's paratrigeminal neuralgia. The association of pain in the eye and forehead with a partial Horner's syndrome (ocular sympathetic paralysis) is known as Raeder's syndrome (66). It may be caused by any lesion bridging the gap between the internal carotid artery, which carries the ocular sympathetic fibers in its wall, and the trigeminal nerve. It may be simulated by disease of the internal carotid wall, such as dissecting aneurysm (71), or by cluster headache in which the same symptom complex recurs episodically.

Gradenigo's syndrome.   The combination of fronto-temporal
pain with an ipsilateral sixth cranial nerve palsy is known as
Gradenigo's syndrome.   It is caused by osteomyelitis or
neoplastic invasion of the apex of the petrous temporal bone.

Inflammation.
Post-herpetic neuralgia is a sequel of shingles in 50% of
patients over the age of 60 years, and in 30% over the age of 40
years.   Herpes Zoster commonly affects the first division of the
trigeminal nerve (ophthalmic herpes) and may thus give rise to
pain in one side of the forehead before, during, and after the
eruption of the rash.

Idiopathic neuralgia.
Trigeminal neuralgia (tic douloureux) is the term applied
to sudden jabbing in the distribution of one or more divisions
of the trigeminal nerve.   It is characteristically precipitated
by trigger factors such as talking or swallowing and may be
elicited by touching specific trigger points around the nose or
lips.   Since 5% of cases affect the first division, trigeminal
neuralgia may be confused with cluster headache and it has
indeed been reported to occur in conjunction with cluster
headache.   Some 2% to 6% of patients with trigeminal neuralgia
have multiple sclerosis, the pain being caused by plaques of
demyelination in the pons at the entry zone of the trigeminal
nerve.   Some, possibly the majority, of the remainder are caused
by compression of the trigeminal nerve in the posterior fossa
(37), usually by the superior cerebellar artery or anterior
inferior cerebellar artery.   Since tic douloureux is such a
distinctive syndrome and there is not yet complete agreement
about its cause, it is best retained in the "idiopathic"
category at present, rather than including it under "compression
of the trigeminal nerve".   Glossopharyngeal neuralgia is a pain
with the same quality as tic douloureux, referred to the ear,
tonsillar fossa and base of the tongue.

Atypical facial pain.
There is one variety of "atypical facial pain" that is so
constant in its characteristics that it warrants consideration
as a separate entity.   It is commonly unilateral, felt deeply in
the nasolabial fold or cheek, and is continuous and boring in
quality.   The pain often dates from a minor dental procedure or
a blow to the face.   Kerr (38) considered that it may be
initiated by a small neuroma at the site of trauma, but may
become a self-perpetuating pain syndrome.

Referred Pain

Eye.
It is rare for ocular conditions other than acute angle
closure glaucoma to refer pain to the head, and aching caused by
acute retrobulbar neuritis or retroorbital tumors is usually

confined to the eye. Imbalance of the extraocular muscles or refractive errors may contribute to tension headache but are not direct sources of pain referral.

Sinuses, nasopharynx.
Acute frontal sinusitis may refer pain to one or both sides of the forehead, while inflammation of the sphenoid or ethmoid sinuses refers pain to the midline. It is uncommon for recurrent headaches to be caused by sinusitis although migraine and cluster headache are often misdiagnosed as such because of the blockage of the nostril that accompanies vascular headaches. Carcinoma of the nasopharynx and sinuses may refer pain to the forehead or temple.

Teeth, temporo-mandibular joints.
Dental caries or apical infection can cause pain in the second and third divisions of the trigeminal nerve which may simulate trigeminal neuralgia. Imbalance of the bite combined with excessive jaw-clenching (bruxism) may cause temporomandibular joint dysfunction with pain radiating from this area to face and temple (Costen's syndrome) (17).

Neck.
Disorders of the upper cervical spine refer pain to the occipital region in the distribution of the second and third cervical roots. Structures implicated include ths synovial joints, intervertebral discs, ligaments and muscles (22) which may be damaged by "whiplash injury" or disease processes such as rheumatoid arthritis. Occipital neuralgia is a paroxysmal jabbing pain in the distribution of the greater or lesser occipital nerves, usually accompanied by diminished sensation or dysaesthesiae of the affected area (32). Lance and Anthony (43) used the term "Neck-Tongue Syndrome" to describe the association of unilateral occipital pain and numbness of the tongue precipitated by sudden rotation of the neck. The syndrome, which first appears in childhood or young adult life, appears to be caused by subluxation of one atlanto-axial joint on extreme rotation, causing pain by stretching the joint capsule (10), and numbness of the tongue by compressing the C-2 ventral ramus which contains proprioceptive fibers from the tongue (43).

Intracranial Causes

Vasodilatation.
Intracranial vessels may dilate and become sensitive to pain in a variety of conditions, giving rise to a bilateral headache which is worse on jolting or head movement. The mechanism is incompletely understood. Causes of such intracranial vascular headache are listed below:
Toxic: for example systemic infections, "hangover" after ingestion of excessive amounts of alcohol, carbon monoxide

poisoning, caffeine withdrawal, foreign protein reactions, drug intoxication.

Metabolic: for example hypoxia, hypoglycemia, hypercapnia. Vasodilator agents such as histamine, nitrites, nitrates, alcohol, monosodium glutamate (MSG) and the inhalation of volatile hydrocarbons used for dry cleaning. The use of MSG in Chinese cooking may give rise to headache as part of the "Chinese Restaurant Syndrome" (60).

Post-concussional: Headache after uncomplicated head injury is uncommon (67), but a comparatively minor blow to the head may precipitate classical migraine, so-called "footballer's migraine" (49).

Post-convulsive: Headache is common after epileptic seizures, probably as a consequence of hypoxia during the fit and a post-ictal increase in cerebral blood flow.

Acute pressor reactions: Headache is a feature in 80% of the hypertensive episodes induced by pheochromocytoma (44, 64). Similar paroxysmal headaches have been reported after the ingestion of foods or drugs containing monoamines by a patient taking monoamine oxidase inhibitors. The resulting pressor response has led to subarachnoid or intracerebral hemorrhage on occasion. The sudden onset of headache at the climax of sexual activity probably has a similar pressor mechanism (40).

Essential hypertension: Sustained hypertension is rarely a cause of headache unless the diastolic pressure exceeds 140 mmHg (2).

Hemodialysis: Headaches experienced by some patients during hemodialysis appear to be of vascular origin and respond to ergotamine (3).

Cerebral vascular disease: Headache, often unilateral, may accompany occlusion of a major cerebral vessel (24), or transient ischemic attacks (30). An intense fronto-temporal headache may follow a day or so after carotid endarterectomy (46, 54).

Meningeal irritation.

Headache and neck rigidity are features of meningeal irritation encountered in subarachnoid hemorrhage, meningitis, encephalitis, and reactions to the injection of foreign substances into the subarachnoid space, for example during myelography or pneumoencephalography.

Traction on, or displacement of, intracranial vessels.

Space-occupying lesions such as hematoma, tumor, or abscess may cause headache by displacing intracranial arteries or by obstructing the flow of cerebrospinal fluid (CSF) through the ventricular system, thus causing internal hydrocephalus.

Raised intracranial pressure may be caused by internal hydrocephalus from such compression of CSF pathways, by aqueduct stenosis, or by obstruction of the foramina of Magendie and Lushka. Communicating hydrocephalus is caused by impairment of circulation of CSF from the basal cisterns through the subarachnoid space to its place of absorption in the superior sagittal sinus. Raised venous pressure, as in emphysema and mediastinal obstruction, or thrombosis of the dominant lateral sinus or superior sagittal sinus ("otitic hydrocephalus") will lead to increased intracranial pressure by reducing CSF absorption. Cerebral edema may be interstitial, surrounding cerebral tumors, or intracellular, after stroke. Patients presenting with headache from raised intracranial pressure without any demonstrable space-occupying lesion, obstruction to CSF pathways or cerebral edema, are said to have "Benign Intracranial Hypertension" (BIH). There are probably a number of causative factors in BIH -- ocult thrombi in the superior sagittal sinus, reduced absorption of CSF by the arachnoid villi, and secondary venous congestion with increase in brain volume (16, 26). The condition may be initiated by head injury, by hormonal factors in obese women, by tetracycline, nalidixic acid, excessive intake of Vitamin A, or cessation of corticosteroid therapy.

Reduced intracranial pressure causes headache by traction on intracranial vessels. It is most commonly caused by leakage of CSF following lumbar puncture.

Benign cough headache.

While headache on coughing is often a symptom of a space-occupying lesion in the posterior fossa, it may persist for years without any structural abnormality being demonstrated. It is possibly caused by a valve-like blockage at the foramen magnum which permits the passage of CSF rostrally during coughing but interferes with the downward or rebound pulsation of CSF (73). Benign exertional headache probably has a different etiology since exercise often triggers vascular headache of the migraine type.

Episodic 'Vascular' Headache

Migraine may be defined as "episodic headache, with or without cerebral disturbance, with intervening periods of relative freedom from headache and without evidence of primary structural abnormality" (41).

Categories of migraine: Migraine may be subdivided as follows by the presence or absence of neurological symptoms:

HEADACHE ASSOCIATED WITH NEUROLOGICAL SYMPTOMS:

Classical migraine.

Episodes in which visual disturbances (or other focal symptoms, such as paresthesias or dysphasia) precede the onset of headache by some 10-60 minutes and fade as the headache develops. "Retinal migraine" is a rare subvariety of classical migraine in which the vision of an eye is impaired or lost as the result of unilateral retinal disturbance, in contrast to the usual visual prodrome which involves one or both half-fields since it originates in the cerebral cortex.

EXTENSION OF NEUROLOGICAL SYMPTOMS INTO THE HEADACHE PHASE:

In some patients, neurological symptoms persist and may increase in severity after the onset of headache. An example is "vertebrobasilar migraine" in which brainstem and cerebellar symptoms or signs precede loss of consciousness that may be brief (syncope) or prolonged ("migraine stupor"). Other variations include "acute confusional migraine" and "hemiplegic migraine"

DEVELOPMENT OF NEUROLOGICAL SYMPTOMS DURING THE HEADACHE PHASE:

On occasions visual or other disturbances, similar in manifestations to the prodromes of classical migraine, may arise during the course of headache. The term "ophthalmoplegic migraine" is applied to an unusual migrainous variant with paresis of ocular motor nerves, particularly the third cranial nerve.

HEADACHE WITHOUT NEUROLOGICAL SYMPTOMS:

Common migraine: Episodic headache, most commonly unilateral and associated with nausea and photophobia, but without overt neurological symptoms and signs, is referred to as "common migraine". Most cases of premenstrual migraine fall into this category. In some patients, headache may extend over the face or pain may be referred to facial structures exclusively ("facial migraine" or "lower half headache").

NEUROLOGICAL SYMPTOMS WITHOUT HEADACHE:

Migraine equivalents: If neurological symptoms evolve and regress like the prodrome of classical migraine without a headache ensuing, the syndrome is called a "migraine equivalent". Such symptoms appearing for the first time in middle-aged or older patients have been termed "transient migrainous accompaniments" (TMAs) by Fisher (25) to distinguish them from thromboembolic transient ischemic attacks (TIAs).

NEUROLOGICAL SIGNS OUTLASTING HEADACHE:

Complicated migraine: Retinal, cerebral or brainstem deficit persisting for more than 24 hours after the cessation of migraine headache or a migraine equivalent is known as "complicated migraine". The term complicated migraine is sometimes used loosely as a synonym for classical migraine but it is preferable to restrict its use to an enduring deficit that is indeed a complication of migraine.

TABLE 3.   Varieties of migraine

Headache associated with neurological symptoms:
Prodromal symptoms: Classical migraine
Symptoms at height of headache:
     Vertebrobasilar migraine
     Migraine stupor
     Acute confusional states of childhood
     Hemiplegic migraine
     Ophthalmoplegic migraine
Headache without neurological symptoms:
     Common migraine
     Facial migraine ("lower half headache")
Neurological symptoms without headache:
     Migraine equivalents
     Transient migrainous accompaniments (TMAs) of middle age
Neurological symptoms and signs outlasting headache:
     Complicated migraine

     Classical migraine. Visual hallucinations of scotomas form
part of the attack in about one-third of all migrainous
patients, commonly appearing as a prodrome to headache. While
some 10% of migrainous patients have experienced "scintillating
scotomas" (fortification spectra, teichopsia), another 25%
describe unformed flashes of light (photopsia) scattered across
one or both visual fields associated with a patchy impairment of
vision which may sometime restrict the peripheral fields,
leaving the patient with tunnel vision. Paresthesias are
reported by 33% (62), while hemiparesis and dysphasia occur in
some 4% of patients (42). The symptoms usually resolve within
the space of an hour as headache develops.
     Vertebrobasilar migraine (basilar artery migraine).
Bickerstaff (5) described 34 of 300 migrainous patients whose
visual disturbance was followed by vertigo, ataxia, dysarthria,
occasionally tinnitus, and paresthesias of lips, tongue and
extremities that lasted up to 45 minutes. The ensuing headache
was commonly occipital. The syndrome was found most often in
adolescent girls and was attributed to ischemia in the
vertebrobasilar circulation as part of the migrainous process.
Bickerstaff (6) also pointed out that impairment or loss of
consciousness occurred at the height of the attack in about
one-third of such patients, presumably because of impaired
vascular supply to the brainstem reticular formation.
Vertebrobasilar migraine may cause episodes of transient global
amnesia (14, 18, 52) and also recurrent vertigo.
     Migraine stupor. Impairment of consciousness is not
uncommon in migraine, usually as a feeling of faintness or
actual syncope as described above. Less commonly, migraine may
be accompanied by stupor or coma. Lee and Lance (45) noted
cases previously reported and described seven patients aged 10-
52 years who had become stuporous for periods varying from half

to five days during attacks of migraine. Associated symptoms and signs included dysarthria, ataxia, incoordination, paresthesias, dilatation of one pupil, and homonymous hemianopia, which suggests that migraine stupor is a severe form of vertebrobasilar migraine.

Acute confusional migraine. An acute confusional state was a feature of migraine attacks in 3.5% of the 500 patients reported by Selby and Lance (62). The condition was described in children by Gascon and Barlow (28), and is probably not uncommon since Ehyai and Fenichel (23) encountered five instances in 100 successive migrainous children seen by them. Disorientation and agitation may be the initial manifestation of migraine, although typical headaches later develop. Confusion lasts for 10 minutes to 20 hours, usually terminating in deep sleep. Attacks may be triggered by relatively minor blows to the head, particularly in children (31), in a manner similar to "footballer's migraine" (4, 49).

Hemiplegic migraine. Hemiparesis associated with migraine has been recognized for more than a century but, with the exception of familial cases, the diagnosis remained uncertain before the advent of cerebral angiography. Whitty (72) described five cases of hemiplegic migraine, four of which were familial. Cerebral angiography in one of these patients precipitated an attack. The literature was reviewed by Bradshaw and Parsons (12) who noted that cerebral angiography in seven reported cases had shown narrowing of internal carotid branches in one instance, and no significant abnormality in the others; angiography had been normal in one of their own patients at the height of hemiplegia. Two of their patients had been unconscious for some days on occasions, thus linking this condition with "migraine stupor", described above. Bradshaw and Parsons widened the definition of hemiplegia migraine to include hemiparesthesias, but this seems to confuse the issue since such sensory symptoms are much more common than hemiparesis. In the familial cases hemiplegic migraine is inherited as a dominant characteristic. "Alternating hemiplegia of childhood", which on occasions may become a quadriparesis with difficulty in swallowing (35), is almost certainly a variant of "hemiplegic migraine".

Ophthalmoplegic migraine is a periodic migrainous headache associated with paralysis of the third cranial nerve, although instances of sixth and fourth nerve palsies have been reported (68). The oculomotor palsy usually comes on at the height of headache or as pain is receding, may persist for weeks after the attack or become permanent after repeated attacks (53). The diagnosis can be made only after exclusion of other conditions such as aneurysm that can compress the third cranial nerve. Walsh and O'Doherty (70) suggested that paresis of the third, fourth, and sixth cranial nerves could be caused either by direct vascular compression or by interference with flow in the vasa nervorum.

Migraine equivalents. Waxing and waning of neurological symptoms over a period of 30-45 minutes in the manner of a prodrome to classical migraine but without headache ensuing is known as a migraine equivalent. A migraine equivalent may appear at any age, most often to patients previously subject to classical migraine. Fisher (25) reported 120 cases of late onset which he termed "Transient Migrainous Accompaniments" with various combinations of visual impairment, paresthesias, paresis and speech disturbance in whom headache was inconspicuous; indeed half had no headache at all after the episode. The diagnosis is made clinically by the "slow march" of symptoms and gradual devolution, quite unlike the abrupt onset of Transient Ischemic Attacks.

Complicated migraine. The term complicated migraine should be reserved for those patients with enduring neurological deficit after the cessation of headache although, in the past, the term has sometimes been used to embrace classical migraine and the migrainous variants considered above, reviewed in detail by Bruyn (13). Pearce and Foster (55) stated that complicated migraine implied "persistent hemiparesis, facial paresis, retinal arterial occlusion or ocular motor palsy in association with an attack of migraine". Bickerstaff (7) as a prelude to his address on "Complicated Migraine", also restricted the term to permanent sequelae of migrainous attacks. The most common visual sequelae are a partial or complete homonymous hemianopia and retinal defects (15), while monocular visual loss may be caused by retinal vascular occlusion, central serous retinopathy or ischemic papillopathy (50). Occipital infarction has been disclosed by CT scanning in patients with visual field defects following migraine (11, 51).

"Abdominal migraine" and vomiting attacks of childhood. Bille (8) found that 20% of migrainous children were subject to paroxysmal abdominal pains compared with 4% of a control group, and regarded such symptoms as a migraine equivalent. Only 1.5% of migrainous patients still suffered abdominal pain at the age of 30 years (9). A past history of vomiting attacks in childhood is obtained in 23% of migrainous patients and 12% of patients with tension headache (42). Recurrent vomiting attacks in adults, often accompanied by abdominal pain or diarrhoea, may be familial and are associated with migraine in one-third of cases (61). There is thus some factual basis for the concept of "abdominal migraine".

Cluster headache.
Cluster headache (periodic migrainous neuralgia) may be defined as a severe unilateral head or facial pain, lasting for minutes or hours, associated commonly with ipsilateral ptosis, lacrimation and blockage of the nostril, usually recurring once or more daily for a period of weeks or months. The term "cluster headache" derives from the tendency for the pain to appear in bouts, separated by intervals of complete freedom (39). The condition has been described previously as ciliary

neuralgia (33, 58), histamine cephalalgia (34), and many more fanciful terms.

Two variations on the theme are recognized. Some patients have all the characteristics of cluster headache except separation into bouts with intervals of freedom. Such patients with regularly recurring attacks without remission are said to suffer from "chronic cluster headache". The second variant has been termed "chronic paroxysmal hemicrania" and is characterized by the frequency of painful episodes, up to 18 recurring in a 24 hour period (63). This variant affects women more often than men (unlike typical cluster headache which affects mostly men), and responds rapidly to treatment with indomethacin.

Tension Headache

Tension headache may be defined as a constant tight or pressing sensation, nearly always bilateral, which may initially be episodic and related to stress but recurs almost daily in its chronic form without regard to any obvious psychological factors. Such headaches are often associated with a mild persisting state of depression. Difficulty arises in classification when tension headache is interspersed with an episodic increase in intensity of headache, associated with nausea and photophobia. The same problem arises when migrainous headache increases in frequency and loses some of its distinctive accompaniments. The term "tension-vascular headache" has been coined to cover these intermediate forms but no clear line can be drawn by clinical judgment or computer analysis between migraine at one end of the idiopathic headache spectrum and chronic tension headache at the other (21). It remains for elucidation of their pathophysiology to determine whether migraine and tension headache are separate entities or whether the associated symptomatology of idiopathic headache depends solely on the frequency and severity of attacks. While excessive muscle contraction may underlie some acute forms of tension headache, the term "muscle contraction headache" is best avoided since studies have not demonstrated any significant difference in electromyographic recordings from the forehead and neck muscles of patients with chronic tension headache and normal controls (1, 47). The mechanism remains obscure but may involve depletion of monoamines in the endogenous pain control system.

Psychogenic Headache

This term is used to describe the association of headache with florid psychiatric disturbance as part of a delusional system. Such headache is a concept of disordered thought processes and appears or disappears with the mental state which engendered it.

REFERENCES

1. Anderson, C. A., and Franks, R. D. (1981): Headache, 21:63.
2. Badran, R. H. Al., Weir, R. J., and McGuiness, J. B. (1970): Scott. Med. J., 15:48.
3. Bana, D. S., Yap, A. U., and Graham, J. R. (1972): Headache, 12:1.
4. Bennett, D. R., Fuenning, S. I., Sullivan, G., and Weber, J. (1980): Am. J. Sports Med., 8:202.
5. Bickerstaff, E. R. (1961): Lancet, 1:15.
6. Bickerstaff, E. R. (1961): Lancet, 2:1057.
7. Bickerstaff, E. R. (1984): In: Progress in Migraine Research, Volume 2, edited by F. Clifford Rose, p. 83. Pitman, London.
8. Bille, B. (1962): Acta Paediatrica, (Suppl. 136), 51:1.
9. Bille, B. (1981): Cephalagia, 1:71.
10. Bogduk, N. (1981): J. Neurol. Neurosurg. Psychiat., 44:202.
11. Bousser, M. G., Baron, J. C., Iba-Zizem, M. T., Comar, D., Cabanis, E., and Castaigne, P. (1980): Stroke, 11:145.
12. Bradshaw, P. and Parsons, M. (1965): Q. J. Med., 34:65.
13. Bruyn, G. W. (1968): In: Handbook of Clinical Neurology, Volume 5, edited by P. J. Vinken and G. W. Bruyn, p. 59. North-Holland, Amsterdam.
14. Caplan, L., Chedru, F., Lhermitte, F., and Mayman, C. (1981): Neurology, 31:1167.
15. Carroll, J. D. (1970): In: Kliniske aspekter i Migraeneforskningen. p. 88. Nordlundes Bogtrykkeri, Copenhagen.
16. Colebatch, J. G., and Lance, J. W. (1983): Aust. J. Ophthalmol., 11:235.
17. Costen, J. B. (1934): Ann. Otol. Rhinol. Lar., 43:1.
18. Crowell, G. F., Stump, D. A., Biller, J., McHenry, L. C., and Toole, J. F. (1984): Arch. Neurol., 41:75.
19. Dornan, T. L., Espir, M. L. E., Gale, E. A. M., Tattersall, R. B., and Worthington, B. S. (1979): J. Neurol. Neurosurg. Psychiat., 42:270.
20. Drummond, P. D., and Lance, J. W. (1984): Clin. Exper. Neurol., 20:93.
21. Drummond, P. D., and Lance, J. W. (1984): J. Neurol. Neurosurg. Psychiat., 47:128.
22. Edmeads, J. (1978): Med. Clins. N. Amer., 62:533.
23. Ehyai, A., and Fenichel, G. M. (1978): Arch. Neurol., 35:368.
24. Fisher, C. M. (1968): In: Handbook of Clinical Neurology, Volume 5, edited by P. J. Vinken and G. W. Bruyn, p. 124. North-Holland, Amsterdam.
25. Fisher, C. M. (1980): Can. J. Neurol. Sci., 7:9.
26. Fishman, R. A. (1984): Arch. Neurol., 41:257.
27. Friedman, A. P., Finley, K. M., Graham, J. R., Kunkle, E. C.; Ostfeld, A. M., and Wolff, W. G. (1962): Arch. Neurol., 6:173.
28. Gascon, G., and Barlow, C. (1970): Pediatrics, 45:628.

29. Gowers, W. R. (1893): In: A Manual of Diseases of the Nervous System, 2nd Edition, Volume 2, p. 856. Blakiston, Philadelphia.
30. Grindal, A. B., and Toole, J. F. (1974): Stroke, 5:603.
31. Haas, D. C., Pineda, G. S., and Lourie, H. (1975): Arch. Neurol., 32:727.
32. Hammond, S. R., and Danta, G. (1978): Clin. Exper. Neurol., 15:258.
33. Harris, W. (1936): Brit. Med. J., 1:457.
34. Horton, B. J.; Mac Lean, A. R., and Craig, W. McK. (1939): Proc. Staff Meet. Mayo Clin., 14:257.
35. Hosking, G. P., Cavanagh, N. P. C., and Wilson, J. (1978): Arch. Dis. Childh., 53:656.
36. Hunt, W. E., Meagher, J. N., Lefever, H. E., and Zeman, W. (1961): Neurology, 11:56.
37. Jannetta, P. J. (1976): Prog. Neurol. Surg., 7:180.
38. Kerr, F. W. L. (1979): In: Advances in Pain Research and Therapy, edited by J. J. Bonica, J. C. Liebeskind, and D. G. Albe-Fessard, p. 283. Raven Press, New York.
39. Kunkle, E. C., Pfieffer, J. B., Jr., Wilhoit, W. M., and Lamrick, L. W. J. (1954): N. Carolina Med. J., 15:510.
40. Lance, J. W. (1976): J. Neurol. Neurosurg. Psychiat., 39:1226.
41. Lance, J. W. (1982): Mechanism and Management of Headache, 4th Edition. Butterworths, London.
42. Lance, J. W., and Anthony, M. (1966): Arch. Neurol., 15:356.
43. Lance, J. W., and Anthony, M. (1980): J. Neurol. Neurosurg. Psychiat., 43:97.
44. Lance, J. W., and Hinterberger, H. (1976): Arch. Neurol., 33:281.
45. Lee, C. H., and Lance, J. W. (1977): Headache, 17:32.
46. Leviton, A., Caplan, L., and Salzman, E. (1975): Headache, 15:207.
47. Martin, P. R., and Mathews, A. M. (1978): J. Psychosom. Res., 22:389.
48. Massey, E. W., and Massey, J. (1979): Headache, 19:339.
49. Matthews, W. B. (1972): Brit. Med. J., 1:326.
50. McDonald, W. I., and Saunders, M. D. (1971): Lancet, 2:531.
51. Moorehead, M. T., Movius, H. J., Moorehead, J. R., Jackson, M.-H. M., and Jackson, J. G. (1979): Southern Med. J., La Grange, 72:821.
52. Olivarius, B. de Fine, and Jensen, T. S. (1979): Headache, 19:335.
53. Pearce, J. (1968): J. Neurol. Sci., 6:73.
54. Pearce, J. (1976): Brit. Med. J., 3:85.
55. Pearce, J. M. S., and Foster, J. B. (1965): Neurology, 15:333.
56. Raskin, N. H., and Knittle, S. C. (1976): Headache, 16:222.
57. Raskin, N. H., and Prusiner, S. (1977): Neurology, 27:43.
58. Romberg, M. H. (1840): A Manual of Nervous Diseases of Man. (trans. E. Sieveking). Sydenham Society, London.

59. Roseman, D. M. (1968): In: Handbook of Clinical Neurology, Volume 5, edited by P. J. Vinken and G. W. Bruyn, p. 375. North-Holland, Amsterdam.
60. Schaumburg, H. H., Byck, R., Gerstl, R., and Mashman, J. H. (1969): Science, 163:826.
61. Scobie, B. A. (1983): Med. J. Australia, 1:329.
62. Selby, G., and Lance, J. W. (1960): J. Neurol. Neurosurg. Psychiat., 23:23.
63. Sjaastad, O., Apfelbaum, R., Caskey, W., Christoffersen, B., Diamond, S., Graham, J., Green, M., Hørven, I., Lund-Roland, L., Medina, J., Rogado, S., and Stein, H. (1980): Uppsala J. Med. Sci., (Suppl. 31), 27.
64. Thomas, J. E., Rooke, E. D., and Kvale, W. F. (1966): JAMA, 197:754.
65. Tolosa, E. (1954): J. Neurol. Neurosurg. Psychiat., 17:300.
66. Toussaint, D. (1968): In: Handbook of Clinical Neurology, Volume 5, edited by P. J. Vinken and G. W. Bruyn, p. 333. North-Holland, Amsterdam.
67. Tubbs, O. N., and Potter, J. M. (1970): Lancet, 2:128.
68. Vijayan, N. (1980): Headache, 20:300.
69. Wadman, B., and Werner, I. (1972): Acta Med. Scandinav., 192:377.
70. Walsh, J. P., and O'Doherty, D. S. (1960): Neurology, 10:1079.
71. West, T. E. T., Davies, R. J., and Kelly, R. E. (1976): Brit. Med. J., 1:818.
72. Whitty, C. W. M. (1953): J. Neurol. Neurosurg. Psychiat., 16:172.
73. Williams, B. (1976): Brain, 99:331.
74. Wolff, H. G. (1963): Headache and Other Head Pain, 2nd Edition. Oxford University Press, New York.

The Management of Headache, edited by F. Clifford Rose. Raven Press, New York © 1988.

EXAMINATION OF THE PATIENT WITH HEADACHE

Michael Anthony, OBE, MD, FRCP, FRACP

Associate Professor, Department of Neurology,
The Prince Henry Hospital, and
The School of Medicine, University of New South Wales,
Sydney, Australia

In the vast majority of cases the correct diagnosis of headache can be made by taking a careful history. Conversely, if no decision can be reached as to the nature of the headache by the time the history is completed, little additional information will be gained by examining the patient. This in no way implies that physical examination is superfluous, as it is necessary not only to suspect but also to actually know that it is negative or, in the case of suspected lesions, that they are in fact present. Further, we should always leave room for the unexpected, no matter how competent we might be in our special field. An outline of the examination of the patient with headache is given in Table 1.

TABLE 1.
    Physical Examination of the Headache Patient

A. Skull
    1. Auscultation - various points
    2. Palpation - tenderness, protruberances, depressions (burr-holes)
B. Temporo-Mandibular Joints
    1. Tenderness on pressure
    2. Limited opening of mouth
    3. Malalignment of bite
C. Neurovascular
    1. Palpation of carotid, temporal, occipital arteries
    2. Auscultation over carotid/vertebral arteries, orbits
D. Cervical Spine
    1. Tenderness over occipital nerves
    2. Sensory examination of scalp
    3. Length of neck - short, long
    4. Flexion, extension, lateral flexion and lateral rotation (active - performed by patient)

E.   Cranial Nerves
     1.   Eyes:
               Visual acuity
               Palpation of eyeballs
               Pupils — unequal or oval
               Cornea — steamy, ciliary injection
               Fundi — optic atrophy or papilledema
     2.   Ears/Hearing:
               External aditory canals
               Type of hearing impairment
     3.   Oculomotor Nerves:
               Congenital/paralytic strabismus
               Ptosis
     4.   Facial movements, sensation and corneal reflexes
F.   Below The Neck
     1.   Limbs — lateralizing weakness or sensory changes
     2.   Reflexes:
               Asymmetry of tendon jerks
               Primitive reflexes
     3.   General:
               Skin lesions, rashes, pigmentation
               Liver, spleen enlargement
               Cardiac lesions — valvular, congenital

The first step in the diagnostic process is to decide whether the particular headache is: (a) acute; (b) subacute; or (c) chronic.

ACUTE HEADACHES

Such headaches commonly have a rapid onset over several minutes or hours, although on occasions this may be sudden or explosive. In the main, acute headaches are severe and frequently they are due to serious underlying pathology.

A simple classification of the causes of acute headache is:
     1.   Intracranial:
         a.   Meningitis/encephalitis
         b.   Subarachnoid hemorrhage
         c.   Subdural hematoma
         d.   Intracranial tumor
     2.   Extracranial:
         a.   Migraine
         b.   Cluster headache
         c.   Post-traumatic headache
         d.   Glaucoma
         e.   Optic neuritis
         f.   Cerebrovasclar insufficiency
     3.   Systemic:
         a.   Hypertension
         b.   Pheochromocytoma
         c.   Reaction to MAO inhibitors

Signs on examination that may be found include:
1.   Signs of meningeal irritation (neck stiffness and a positive Kernig's sign), with or without depression of consciousness   -   meningitis,   encephalitis,   subarachnoid hemorrhage, intracranial tumor.
2.   Depression of consciousness without signs of meningeal irritation - subdural hematoma, intracranial tumor.
3.   Ocular signs - glaucoma, optic neuritis, cluster headache.
4.   Hypertension   -   essential   hypertension, pheochromocytoma, adverse reaction to MAO inhibitors, raised intracranial pressure (tumor, subdural hematoma).

A decision regarding the nature of the headache must be made immediately. If doubt exists, the patient should be admitted to hospital.

SUBACUTE HEADACHES

Headaches which escalate over several days or weeks, in a patient who has not suffered headaches previously or had experienced them only occasionally, belong in this category. It is this group of patients that harbor potentially the most serious causes of headache. These include:
a.   Subdural hematoma
b.   Temporal arteritis
c.   Cerebral abscess
d.   Tumor
e.   Intracranial sinus thrombosis
f.   Benign intracranial hypertension

The signs on examination may include:
1.   Papilledema, can be produced by any of the above causes except temporal arteritis.
2.   Lateralizing signs (e.g., asymmetric reflexes) in subdural hematoma, cerebral abscess, and tumor.
3.   Fever, in cerebral abscess, temporal arteritis.
4.   Raised ESR in temporal arteritis.
5.   Depression of consciousness or confusion, in subdural hematoma, cerebral abscess, tumor.

Patients with any of the above signs should be investigated with a CT brain scan, full blood count and ESR. These investigations will identify the nature of the intracranial lesion, or of the arterial inflammation in temporal arteritis. The value of EEG and cerebral angiography has now diminished with the advent of computer scanning.

CHRONIC HEADACHES

Headaches which have been consistent for two or more years and are not associated with any neurological signs are almost certainly of the migraine or tension variety. They require no special investigations unless atypical and fail to respond to preventive treatment.

SPECIAL INVESTIGATIONS

These are rarely necessary, as in the majority of cases a full history and clinical examination are adequate for diagnosis. Where doubt exists the investigation of choice is a CT brain scan, which has effectively replaced plain X-rays of the skull, angiography, pneumoencephalography and ventriculography. These procedures, apart from cerebral angiography, are now used only in exceptional circumstances. Angiography is indicated in patients with suspected cerebral aneurysm and in those with cerebrovascular insufficiency, where it is the investigation of choice. Lumbar puncture should be performed only when the presence of intracranial tumor has been excluded by CT brain scan and in order to confirm the presence of meningitis, encephalitis or subarachnoid hemorrhage. A full blood count and ESR are necessary to exclude temporal arteritis, where a leucocytosis and a high ESR confirm the diagnosis. A summary of investigations of the headache patient is given in Table 2 (see also next Chapter).

TABLE 2.

Investigations for Headache

A.   Probably Unnecessary:
    1.   Skull and Chest X-ray
    2.   Electroencephalogram (EEG)
    3.   Radionuclide Brain Scan
B.   Necessary and Informative
    1.   CT Brain Scan
    2.   Blood Count, ESR
    3.   Carotid Artery Ultrasound (Doppler)
    4.   Facial Thermography
    5.   Digital Subtraction Angiography
C.   Inpatient Investigations for:
    1.   Infections - CSF Examination
    2.   Surgical Lesions:
              Contrast Studies
              Angiogram
              Pneumoencephalogram
              Myelogram

It is obvious from the above that the more acute the headache the greater the need for speedy diagnosis. If this cannot be arrived at quickly, it is best to refer the patient to the appropriate hospital unit or medical specialist for expert opinion and appropriate treatment.

The Management of Headache, edited
by F. Clifford Rose. Raven Press,
New York © 1988.

DIFFERENTIAL DIAGNOSIS OF HEADACHE

K. J. Zilkha

There can be few symptoms with such a vast number of causes as headache. Whether the patient presents with a long or short history, to a general practitioner or physician, there are no substitutes to a good history taking and full examination.

The diagnosis may be all too obvious -- but even a long history of classical migraine, when there has been a change in the pattern of headache, may herald the possibility of another cause for the symptoms:

MD had a ten year history of unilateral headaches with nausea and occasional vomiting. He developed blurring of vision, had papilledema and a hemangioblastoma of the cerebellum was removed at the National Hospital, Queen Square. Three months later his migraine returned.

MB gave a twenty year history of migraine. She developed a partial 3rd nerve palsy on the same side as the headache, and an angiogram confirmed the diagnosis of a posterior communicating aneurysm, which was later successfully clipped. She continued to have migraine attacks.

It is relatively easy to make a very long list of possible causes of headache. Indeed it may be more difficult to list what conditions may not be associated with headaches.

Morning headache, with nausea and perhaps vomiting is worthy of concern, as it may indicate raised intracranial pressure, and papilledema may be a late rather than early development.

Constant headache and perhaps tenderness may indicate local pathology, sinus infection, glaucoma and of course temporal arteritis.

Dental pain may not always be self evident -- and the pain may be referred, sooner or later, to the head.

Temporomandibular joint arthritis, and malocclusion are not uncommon, and may be responsible for a good deal of constant pain in the head. Jaw and teeth clenching may be remarked upon by other members of the family.

Cervical spondylosis may be the cause but when it is so common, particularly over the age of 40, can we be sure it is the sole explanation?

Hypertension is obviously an important physical sign, but it is the intermittent rise in blood pressure, certainly at the beginning, which may be missed and yet may be the only clue to the presence of a pheochromocytoma.

Benign intracranial hypertension, typically in young obese women, is a diagnosis of exclusion. Papilledema is usually present. There may also be obscurations of vision, diplopia and vomiting. A CT showing small ventricles, and the raised cerebrospinal fluid pressure on lumbar puncture confirm the diagnosis.

A vascular malformation may be associated with symptomatic migraine, but it is cerebral aneurysm which can cause difficulty in diagnosis and may not be demonstrated by CT scanning.

Of course in sheer numbers, headache due to anxiety and depression remains all too common, and muscle tension headache runs it a close second.

Atypical facial pain usually has a definite depressive component by the time it is seen by the neurologist. It is obviously a misnomer, for one begins to recognize its characteristics, with unilateral, sometimes bilateral, facial pain accompanying the headache. I have not been convinced of the presence of a single trigger factor -- although in recent years I have recognized a subdivision affecting women who earn a living by sewing, and I have termed it "machinist headache". It nearly always responds to antidepressant therapy.

Trigeminal neuralgia, "tic douloureux" is so characteristic, with its 5th nerve distribution, trigger factors of touch, talking and eating and its periodicity, that there can be little reason to mistake the diagnosis. It is more common over the age of 60. When it occurs in a younger person, there is always the possibility of a structural lesion, such as a neurofibroma or multiple sclerosis, particularly if there are physical signs.

Migraine is a special kind of headache. I think that Gowers' description (2) still remains the most elegant: "Migraine is an affection characterized by paroxysmal nervous disturbances, of which headache is the most constant element. The pain is seldom absent and may exist alone, but it is commonly accompanied by nausea and vomiting, and it is often preceded by some sensory disturbance especially by some disorder of the sense of sight. The symptoms are frequently one-sided and from this character of the headache the name is derived."

Compare that with the definition as suggested by the Ad Hoc Committee on Classification of Headache (1). This defines migraine as: "Recurrent attacks of headache, widely varied in intensity, frequency and duration. The attacks are commonly unilateral at onset, are usually associated with anorexia and sometimes with nausea and vomiting; and some are preceded by or associated with conspicuous sensory, motor, and mood disturbances, and are often familial."

But one can go further, and as well as classical migraine and common migraine, we can list migraine accompagnee, ophthalmoplegic and hemiplegic migraine and of course abdominal migraine in childhood and young adult life. It has long been debated whether uncomplicated hypertension ever gives rise to headache. Well it does, and what is more it is relieved by hypotensive treatment. Migraine complicated by hypertension may be unresponsive to treatment that does not also lower the blood pressure! I am not going to discuss management or treatment further, but I would like to highlight some features that have guided me over the years.

Daily headache is hardly ever due to simple or common or classical migraine. I have encountered it in ergotamine dependent headache, in those patients with migraine who regularly take ergotamine. I have also seen it in vascular headache, associated with administration of The Pill, dietary triggered migraine, and of course migraine complicated by tension and depression.

Post-herpetic neuralgia may occasionally present with only a few blisters of herpes zoster to indicate the true nature of the unilateral pain.

Unilateral headache may accompany or precede carotid or cerebral arterial occlusions, and of course cerebral hemorrhage. Head trauma, with or without litigation, may be associated with protracted headache, and usually there is no demonstrable abnormality on X-rays or CT scanning. It is not unusual for depression and loss of confidence to complicate the clinical picture.

We have all experienced headache in association with a feverish illness, but much more severe is the pain in bacterial and viral meningitis, and rickettsial illness. One sees hangover headache socially, but I suppose the sufferer is hardly likely to miss the diagnosis unless again it is complicated by an injury.

Drug causes of headache can be quite difficult to pinpoint. Unless the association is clearcut, and early in onset, then it may be missed. Everyone is now fully aware of the association of monoamine oxidase inhibitors and headache in those foolish enough not to follow advice and exclude those foods rich in amines.

Simple investigations are not usually rewarding, and X-rays of the skull can, but rarely do, demonstrate the decalcification of the sella to indicate chronic raised intracranial pressure, or the shift of the calcified pineal, to indicate the lateralization of a space occupying lesion. An erythrocyte sedimentation rate estimation is mandatory in those over 60 with headache, but temporal arteritis can occur below 60, as does polymyalgia rheumatica, and the ESR may be little raised, and one must go on to temporal artery biopsy and the administration of steroids.

I find that X-rays of the cervical spine so often show spondylosis that it would be difficult to say that there is a definite causal relationship.

A chest X-ray is always informative, but not always of direct relevance to the problem.

CT scanning has become the routine investigation all neurologists feared that it would -- so now we have to take a history after someone else has already noted a negative scan! That said, it is still the experience of us all that we have picked up "silent" lesions, when the scan was done for another purpose. In my own case, recently I have seen a young woman with tension headache who needed a lot of reassurance, and whose scan showed a very small colloid cyst of the third ventricle with normal lateral ventricles. Another patient, a serving officer presented with vertigo, and had a small parasagittal meningioma! Some units claim 85% abnormalities in their scan results. I think this is exceptional, and we are all prepared to see many normal scans in the course of reassurance.

I am not going to discuss invasive investigation techniques; they come in later Chapters and they do not contribute to the strict differential diagnosis, but to the further management of the condition.

When a patient presents with a headache, the doctor has a chance of practising the full art and science of medicine.

REFERENCES

1. Friedman, A. P., Finley, K. M., Graham, J. R., Kunkle, E. C.; Ostfeld, A. M., and Wolff, W. G. (1962): Arch. Neurol., Chicago, 6:173.
2. Gowers, W. R. (1893): In: A Manual of Diseases of the Nervous System, 2nd Edition, Blakiston, Philadelphia.

The Management of Headache, edited
by F. Clifford Rose. Raven Press,
New York © 1988.

SPECIAL INVESTIGATIONS IN MIGRAINE

K. M. A. Welch, MD

Chairman, Department of Neurology, Henry Ford Hospital,
2799 West Grand Boulevard, Detroit, Michigan 48202, U.S.A.

J. A. Helpern, Michael Chopp, and James R. Ewing

Department of Neurology, Henry Ford Hospital,
2799 West Grand Boulevard, Detroit, Michigan 48202, U.S.A.

Special investigations by definition are all testings other
than routine laboratory clinical pathology, electrophysiology
and radiological procedures available in a contemporary clinical
neurological center. For the most part, the diagnosis of
migraine is made on clinical history and examination, with
laboratory testing performed only if metabolic or structural
disease is suspected. In most practices, the number of migraine
patients that require partial or complete further evaluation
with EEG, evoked responses, CT and arteriography is small and
limited largely to patients with complicated symptoms and signs
of focal neurological deficit associated with an otherwise
typical migraine headache. Nevertheless this group is
significant in size and at increased risk for invasive
procedures such as arteriography. The groups of patients that
would benefit from a definitive or diagnostic test for migraine
include: (i) classical or complicated migraine; (ii) atypical
vascular headache; (iii) initial episode of headache,
particularly of late age onset; (iv) migraine equivalents; (v)
late onset migraine equivalents (Fisher); and (vi) research
patients.

To date no definitive diagnostic test has been derived,
despite extensive research investigations utilizing biochemical
and physiological approaches that have generally included
biochemical studies of blood elements or CSF, thermography and
measurements of cerebral blood flow (CBF). Positron Emission
Tomograph (PET), Magnetic Resonance Imaging (MRI) and NMR
spectroscopy are the most recent techniques with as yet
unestablished findings.

A review of the most established research studies performed
to date follows. The findings are evaluated for their
specificity as a putative diagnostic test for migraine, but it

is concluded that at this time a specific diagnostic test does
not exist, although there is the promise of NMR spectroscopy in
the future diagnosis of migraine.

PLATELET STUDIES

The observation of increased 5'hydroxyindole-acetic acid
(5-HIAA) excretion in urine obtained from patients during
migraine headache was the first indication that altered
5-hydroxytryptamine (5-HT) metabolism might contribute to
migraine (51). This was followed by the study of Anthony et al.
who confirmed that significant changes occurred in platelet 5-HT
throughout the prodromal and headache phases of the migraine
attack (1). These studies focused attention on the possibility
that abnormal function of platelets may be an important factor
in this condition's etiology. In fact, it has been claimed that
migraine is a systemic disorder of platelet function (20).

Aggregation Responses

Drs. Hilton and Cumings were the first scientists to report
increased platelet aggregation in response to 5-HT in patients
with migraine (24). Patients free of migraine and drugs for at
least three days gave high values for aggregation responses
after preincubation with 5-HT itself, aggregation being measured
by the Born turbidometric method (5). Patients free of headache
but on methysergide consistently showed much lower aggregation
responses after preincubation. 5-HT-induced platelet
aggregation is dependent on the availability of uptake sites on
the platelets. When the uptake site is empty, aggregation can
occur, but if the uptake site is already occupied by a 5-HT
molecule, aggregation cannot take place. Hilton et al. showed
that the aggregation response of human platelets to 5-HT was
inversely proportional to the content of 5-HT in whole blood.
In their study, patients with migraine had platelets which
aggregated more readily after preincubation with 5-HT than
controls, which implied that the platelet uptake sites accepted
5-HT less readily, or were less capable of retaining 5-HT than
normal subjects. It was postulated that because aggregation
responses of the platelets were dependent on the state of sites
for the transfer of 5-HT through the plasma membrane, these
transfer sites on the membranes of migraine patients were
abnormal.

The above studies have been substantiated over the years by
other workers who have studied active uptake mechanisms for 5-HT
into platelets. Malmgren et al. (32) showed reduced accumulation
of 5-HT in platelets from migraine patients when samples were
studied between attacks. Launay et al. (30) found the Michaelis
constant (Km) and maximum rate of uptake (V-max) of 5-HT into
platelets were reduced during a migraine attack. The following
table shows that when patients had a migraine attack within five
days of the study, there was a significantly lower value of

V-max for 5-HT uptake than in controls. There was no significant change in Km.

TABLE 1.   Platelet 5-HT uptake in five patients
             tested with and without recent migraine.[a]

Attack Time:	Km	V-max (pmoles/10^8) platelets/min
Within 5 days	0.51 ± 0.13	22.2 ± 1.7 (N.S.)($p > 0.02$)
No attack within	0.46 ± 0.04	33.7 ± 3.5

[a]Adapted from Carroll et al. (8).

Active uptake of 5-HT has been further investigated (59) using tritiated ^3H imipramine which putatively labels recognition sites on the platelet surface mediating 5-HT uptake. Binding capacity was reduced in classical migraineurs between attacks and to a more marked degree in males than females. The capacity for uptake was further reduced in migraineurs shortly after an attack. This series of carefully performed studies led to the conclusion that the behavior of platelets in regard to 5-HT function was altered in patients with migraine. The question remains whether the findings are due to a primary abnormality of serotonergic function or secondary to some plasmatic factor.

Other Indices of Platelet Aggregation

Kalendovsky et al., using screen filtration techniques, found platelet hyperaggregability to adenosine diphosphate (ADP), 5-HT and epinephrine in migraine patients, particularly those with complicated migraine (26). In a careful study performed by Couch et al., who applied optical density methods, platelet aggregation was tested in 46 patients with migraine matched by age, sex and race with 46 controls (9). Migraine patients demonstrated platelet hyperaggregability manifested by a lower threshold for the platelet release reaction and an increased platelet adhesiveness following the aggregation. These results were confirmed in a smaller series of experiments by Deshmukh and Meyer (11). Couch and Hassanein (9) also showed that there was no correlation of this platelet hyperaggregability with the severity of migraine or occurrence of associated neurological symptoms suggesting that hyperaggregability is a concomitant feature of the migraine syndrome, but not dependent on the occurrence of the actual headache. Jones et al. have been unable to find an abnormality of aggregation to either ADP or epinephrine in their patients with classical migraine (25), although they did not study platelet release phenomena or disaggregation of platelets. Welch et al., using the Born technique, studied the threshold for the platelet's release reaction (59), and found that patients with complicated migraine had a markedly increased aggregation to epinephrine but significantly less to ADP. Common migraine patient showed no such changes. However, when disaggregation responses to ADP were examined, migraine patients did show a reduced disaggregability to ADP which was markedly accentuated in those with complicated features.

Microemboli Index

Wu et al. (62) devised a technique for the quantitation of platelet aggregates using a differential platelet count ratio. These ratios have shown increased aggregation of circulating platelet microemboli in patients with transient ischemic attacks, myocardial infarction and acute peripheral arterial insufficiency. Increased circulating microemboli have been found both between attacks and during the headache phase of migraine (11), and these results have been confirmed by others, but it needs to be emphasized that the number of circulating aggregates does not change during a migraine attack. Furthermore, the number of aggregates was not elevated in patients with complicated migraine in between attacks.

Several laboratories have reported elevated platelet adhesiveness in migraine patients (11,59), but this adhesiveness does not consistently change during the headache attack compared to in between attacks.

When the results of in vitro aggregation studies, circulating microemboli levels and platelet adhesiveness are assessed together, it can be concluded that migraine patients have hyperaggregability of platelets as reflected by responses to particular in vitro aggregating agents, ADP and epinephrine. In addition, platelets have reduced ability to disaggregate once aggregation has taken place due to abnormally high adhesiveness. Complicated migraine patients have much "stickier" platelets with even greater adhesiveness and the ability to form even tighter aggregates once platelet microemboli form. This quality alone might be an important factor in the difference between clinical symptomatology of common and classic migraine since the formation of tighter platelet aggregates during a migraine attack might be expected to produce more significant occlusion of the cerebral microvasculature leading to ischemic neurological deficit.

Adenine Nucleotide Content of Platelets

5-HT normally present in blood is stored in platelets as high molecular weight aggregates with the adenine nucleotides ATP and ADP. When ATP, ADP and AMP were estimated during various phases of the migraine attack, no statistical difference was found before, during or after the headache (2), but later studies suggested that platelets of migraine patients contain significantly more ADP and total adenine nucleotides than normal platelets (43). These findings were confirmed in Hanington's laboratory; ADP and ATP were elevated in platelets obtained from patients with classical migraine (21). The significance of these findings is uncertain but possibly involves 5-HT uptake into the platelet since the process of uptake is an active one and is proportional to ATP content. These studies are perhaps more significant for demonstrating again that there are differences in platelet behavior in migraineurs when compared to normal controls.

Platelet Releasing Factor

A releasing factor in plasma has been postulated to cause a decrease in platelet 5-HT during the migraine attack. Anthony and Lance (4) were the first to explore this phenomenon and the results of this study are shown in Table 2.

TABLE 2. 5-HT content (μg/10^9 of headache-free platelets when incubated with platelet-poor plasma or its infiltrate, from headache-free periods and from the migraine attack

	Number of Patients	Headache Free Pre-Headache	Headache	Headache Free Post-Headache	Number of Patients Showing a Decrease
Platelet-poor plasma	30	0.48	0.38	0.50	18
Filtrate of platelet-poor plasma	16	0.41	0.34		16

Thirty patients were investigated and 24 showed a significant fall in plasma 5-HT during the migraine attack. The 5-HT content of platelets, when incubated with plasma taken from patients during the attack, was significantly lower than when incubation took place during a headache-free period. From these studies, Anthony postulated that there is a factor in plasma which releases 5-HT from the platelet and that its molecular weight is 50×10^3 or less. This tends to exclude most plasma proteins and antigen antibody complexes, but raises the possibility of fatty acids such as prostaglandins, polypeptides or other monoamines.

These results have been confirmed by Muck-Seler et al. who studied 24 migrainous patients and found a significant fall in platelet 5-HT when platelets from blood collected during headache-free intervals were incubated with platelet poor plasma

taken from other migrainous patients during an attack (36,56).
This was not seen in plasma taken during a headache-free period.
Moreover, plasma from migraine patients taken during an attack
did not elicit 5-HT release from platelets of healthy controls.
This would tend to accentuate the importance of the demonstrable
differences in platelet aggregability between migraineurs and
controls found in other studies.

Anthony has searched for his factor but currently all
evidence for its presence has been indirect (56). He also
postulated that free fatty acids may be involved in the process.
In support of this, he measured significant elevations of total
plasma free fatty acids in eight of ten patients, and selective
elevations of stearic and palmitic acid in nine of ten and
elevations of oleic and linoleic acid in all ten.

Evidence for a Platelet Release Reaction During Migraine Attacks

When an aggregating agent is added to platelets, they
undergo a shape change followed by aggregation. If the stimulus
is strong enough, a release reaction takes place by which the
stored contents of platelet granules are released and the
platelet aggregation cascade progresses. Gawel et al. have
studied this platelet release reaction in migraine (14). In
particular, they measured beta-thromboglobulin (B-TG), a
specific release product of the platelet. The mean level of
B-TG did not change in between migraine attacks but doubled
during an attack. D'Andrea et al. (10) found a significant
elevation in plasma B-TG and Platelet Factor 4 (PF4) levels in
classical migraine, but only B-TG elevation in common migraine.

Platelet Enzyme Studies

A major enzyme involved in the metabolism of biogenic
amines is monoamine oxidase (MAO). Based on differential
sensitivity to inhibition by chlorgyline and l-deprenyl, two
catalytically active forms MAO-A and MAO-B, have been
identified. Noradrenaline and 5-HT are usually deaminated by
MAO-A whereas benzylamine and phenylethylamine have a high
affinity for the MAO-B. Dopamine and tyramine are metabolized
by both. High amounts of MAO-B have been detected in human
platelets (35).

Patients with dietary provoked migraine appear to have an
increased sensitivity to tyramine by virtue of a deficiency in
MAO. Several studies have reported MAO-B activity to be
significantly lower in patients with migraine (6,46,47,50), but
not all studies have been entirely supportive of this finding.
Glover et al. observed decreased MAO activity in classical
migraine in males but not in females or patients with common
migraine (17). Thomas found no difference between patients with
classical migraine and controls (55). A transitory decrease in
platelet MAO activity has been described in migraine patients

during a migraine attack in both males and females (18), although there appeared to be no obvious relationship between MAO characteristics and headache frequency or time since the last headache attack. More recently Waldenlind et al. (57) have confirmed that V-max values for MAO-B activity are significantly lower in migraine patients than controls. They also found a more significant thermolability of the enzyme and suggested that their findings represent constitutionally different enzyme properties in migraineurs than normal controls. However, an endogenous MAO inhibitor in plasma could account for the findings.

From the evidence reviewed in the previous pages, two viewpoints emerge that the migraine syndrome is a primary disorder of the platelet or it is secondary. The summary evidence for a primary disorder is obtained from the differences in platelet membrane uptake for 5-HT found in between attacks, hypersensitivity of in vitro aggregation responses, increased platelet adhesiveness, altered platelet MAO-B activity and differences in adenine nucleotide content. The platelet membrane differences also may be a reflection of a general membrane abnormality genetically expressed in the platelet. Possibly the same membrane abnormality is expressed in the neuron and could be the basis for a primary CNS site of origin for the attack.

The concept of the platelet abnormality being secondary is supported by: (i) a documented but unidentified releasing factor; (ii) conflicting evidence that aggregation responses are different in between attacks; (iii) insufficient experimental details in reported studies to be confident that the abnormal platelet function measured in between attacks is in fact not a residual finding from a secondary disorder of platelet dysfunction occasioned by the attack itself; (iv) the postulated presence of a circulating plasmatic factor that might be expressing its presence by altering platelet function (e.g., reduced MAO-B activity); (v) the effect of stress and pain on platelet function perhaps manifest through plasmatic factors or neurogenically mediated circulatory responses which secondarily alter platelet function during the attack and for some undetermined period thereafter; and (vi) the circulating platelets may become activated as they pass through oligemic/ischemic brain during a migraine attack.

The body of information obtained so far does not provide convincing evidence that migraine is a primary platelet disorder, and none of the special investigations alone can provide a definitive diagnosis of migraine. Probably the most convincing and reproducible changes are the fall in platelet 5-HT and release of B-TG and PF-4 in classic and common migraine.

CSF STUDIES

It has been proposed that pain supersensitivity related to depletion of 5-HT in the CNS is of fundamental importance in the migraine syndrome (49). Evidence that the serotonergic system has an inhibitory influence on central perception of pain can be gained from both animal and clinical studies (22,48), but findings from the few reported studies concerning the 5-HT metabolite 5-HIAA in CSF from migraine patients have been too inconsistent to confirm depletion of CNS 5-HT during a migraine attack (27,41).

Gamma-aminobutyric acid (GABA) and 3'-5' cyclic adenosine monophosphate (cAMP) have been studied in CSF of patients with migraine because of the putative involvement of these two substances in both cerebral energy metabolism and the electrochemical synaptic transmission events of Spreading Depression (58). GABA was measured in CSF obtained from patients during a migraine headache, and control studies were performed in CSF obtained by a diagnostic spinal tap during headache-free intervals in patients with muscle contraction headache and migraine. cAMP was also measured in CSF obtained from migraine patients when a lumbar puncture was performed during or within 48 hours of vascular headaches of migraine type. GABA was analyzed by an enzymatic, fluorimetric assay and cAMP was analyzed by protein binding assay. GABA was undetectable in controls because of low sensitivity of the assay, but eight patients with migraine of classical and common type were studied and GABA was detected in all cases. In 13 patients, the mean cAMP value was also elevated during or within 48 hours of a migraine attack when compared to controls.

Several studies have indicated that the changes in cranial blood flow during migraine involve a decrease in CBF during the prodromal phase and an increase in the headache. Since the biochemical changes during migraine are similar to those also observed in patients with occlusive cerebral vascular disease of recent onset (58), it seems to be a strong possibility that the elevations in CSF, GABA and cAMP occur secondarily to transient cerebral ischemia. The mechanisms whereby these substances are elevated in ischemic brain itself have not been defined, but could be related to disturbance of cerebral energy metabolism provoked by ischemia. The cAMP findings may have particular relevance to the development of headache associated with a migraine attack inasmuch as increased CSF concentrations of lactate also have been found to occur at this time (53). This is probably due to a shift towards anerobic cerebral glycolysis and development of tissue lactic acidosis during migraine headache. cAMP is known to have controlling effects at different steps of the glycogenolytic and glycolytic cycles and its elevation may therefore be a factor which promotes tissue lactic acidosis. Cerebral lactic acidosis may increase cerebral blood flow and possibly headache (58).

Some experimental studies have demonstrated elevated cAMP and GABA in brain tissue in animal models of Spreading Depression (28,42). Spreading Depression is a currently popular concept to explain the hemodynamic and metabolic changes observed in the migraine attack. Thus, elevation of CSF, GABA, and cAMP does not confirm hypoxic ischemia during a migraine attack, but nevertheless, although the evidence is indirect, it does confirm central metabolic shifts. As a definitive test for migraine, however, these CSF findings are unsatisfactory by virtue of similar changes due to cerebral ischemia.

Thermography

Lance et al. were among the first to study migraine patients with thermography (29), and found that cranial skin temperature decreased ipsilateral to the headache suggesting shunting of blood to deeper cranial structures during the migraine attack. In contrast, cluster headache patients develop a cold spot followed by a hot spot localized to the site of pain, usually periorbital.

Whereas thermography is of interest in indirectly monitoring shifts in cranial flow during migraine, the technique is not definitive because vascular changes of multifactorial etiology cause similar changes.

Cerebral Blood Flow Studies

In the 1940's, Wolff introduced the concept that the aura of classical migraine is produced by vasoconstriction, and the headache is an "epiphenomenon" resulting from neurogenic vasodilatation of the pain-sensitive extracranial vessels in response to this ischemic incident (61). In recent years, closer study of CBF has been achieved by 133-Xenon intracarotid injection or inhalation followed by tracer detection (12,16,19,34,37-39,44,45,52,53). Serendipitous use of these methods during a migraine attack has confirmed significant changes in CBF. Mean reductions of 23% in CBF have been observed during an aura (12,13,16,19,34,37-39,44,45,52,53,58). During the headache, CBF has been measured at over 150% normal (53). The prodromal oligemia may be focal or spread to involve the asymptomatic cortex (16,34,53). The findings of cerebral angiography at this time have been reported as normal, with the exception of occasional abnormal filling of the basilar artery (34,61). In general, a global hyperemia develops during the headache phase (12,16,19,34,37,38,53). Currently this vasodilatation is thought to be a metabolic phenomenon induced by local lactic acidosis and hypoxia (12,13,53,58). The global hyperemia may persist over 48 hours beyond resolution of symptoms, or continue only in the neurologically-symptomatic cortex (19,34,62). Mechanisms of these blood flow changes are unknown. In addition to the concept of initial vasospasm followed by metabolically induced hyperemia, an extracranial-intracranial steal mechanism has been proposed to allow for the extracranial vasodilatation frequently recorded during an attack as well as the intracranial oligemia/ischemia (60). The concept of a reduction in CBF secondary to neuronal inhibition caused by Spreading Depression has recently re-emerged following the observation of a spreading cerebral oligemia during the prodrome of a migraine attack (39). The CBF increase recorded during headache also has been attributed by some to neuronal activation caused by pain (12,19).

CEREBRAL METABOLISM

To date, there has been no direct evidence that cerebral metabolism is altered during an attack of migraine; CBF studies provide only indirect support. Two techniques for the non-invasive measurement of cerebral metabolism in man have emerged in the last few years, the most recent being Nuclear Magnetic Resonance spectroscopy, and there is greater potential for studying migraine mechanisms with this technique.

31-P Topical Magnetic Resonance

Nuclear Magnetic Resonance (NMR) promises to revolutionize investigational medicine, not only because of its potential to image anatomical structures within the human body with exquisite resolution far beyond the capability of the CT scan, but because of its capacity using the same principles to measure metabolic function in the organs and structures that are imaged. Topical Magnetic Resonance (TMR) is a particular technique that employs NMR principles to identify biochemical signals in a focus of interest in an anatomical structure. Although many organs can be studied, this discussion will be limited to the TMR of brain. With this technique, spectra of high energy phosphate compounds can be obtained from a human brain by a totally non-invasive approach. Since these compounds are the essentials of brain energetics, they are fundamental for understanding normal brain function and many brain diseases.

We have employed the use of a TMR 32-600 Oxford Research Instruments superconducting magnet with a 70 cm bore at 1.89 Tesla field strength. Patients are placed inside the magnet with the brain imaged, utilizing a proton signal and employing a 2D-FT with slice technique. A sensitive spot is created by shaping the magnet field using separate head coils. The structure of anatomical interest obtained from the brain image is then positioned in the center of the sensitive spot using stereotactic procedures. A surface coil placed on the head close to the region of interest is then employed for pulse-acquisition of the 31-P signal from the area of interest. The result is a spectrum of phosphate compounds obtained from an approximately 4 cm diameter volume of the brain. Note that important information can be obtained from this spectrum in terms of energy status of human brain. Since the values for the phosphate compounds cannot be quantified precisely by virtue of the unavailability of tissue for in vitro biochemical analysis in man, emphasis is placed on ratios, particularly the phosphocreatine/ATP ratio and the inorganic phosphate/phosphocreatine ratio, both of which provide a good indication of dynamic shifts in energy metabolism. In addition, by measuring the position of the inorganic phosphate peak in the spectrum relative to phosphocreatine, it is possible to calculate intracellular pH.

By utilizing the techniques described we can also obtain information from the extracranial tissues, particularly temporal muscle. Head spectra contrasts with brain spectrum, particularly in regard to the large phosphodiester peak and the much greater phosphocreatine peak contributed by muscle. Table 3 shows the relative values for ratios in the head compared to brain in normal young clinical volunteers. Thus, during any one attack of migraine, it is possible to measure energy metabolic status in both the extracranial and intracranial structures.

A major advantage of the technique is that it is possible o scan dynamically for shifts in energy metabolic status for as ong as the patient can remain immobile in the magnet.

Thus far we have studied established human ischemic infarction preliminary to studying dynamic observations in progressing stroke and migraine. Success in detecting ischemic metabolic perturbations in man promises well for future migraine studies. Currently we are collecting data in cluster headache patients used also as pain controls. No significant changes in energy metabolism have been obtained in a small number of patients.

TABLE 3.

	PCr:Beta-ATB	Pi:PCr
Head	1.30 - 1.39	0.15 - 0.34
Brain	0.96 - 0.71	0.67
Stroke		
Ipsilateral	1.04 - 0.19	0.58
Contralateral	0.72 - 0.34	0.72

REFERENCES

1. Anthony, M., Hinterberger, H., and Lance, J. W. (1967): Arch. Neurol., 16:544.
2. Anthony, M., Hinterberger, H., and Lance, J. W. (1969): Res. Clin. Stud. Headache, 2:29.
3. Anthony, M., and Lance, J. W. (1968): Med. J. Aust., 1:56.
4. Anthony, M., and Lance, J. W. (1975): In: Modern Topics in Migraine, edited by J. Pearce, pp. 107-123, Chapter 11. William Heinemann Medical Books Ltd., London.
5. Born, G. V. R. (1962): Nature, London, 194:927.
6. Bussone, G., Giovannini, P., Boiardi, A., and Boeri, R. (1977): Eur. Neurol., 15:157.
7. Carlson, L. A., Ekelund, L. G., and Oro, L. (1968): Acta Med. Scandinav., 183:423.
8. Carroll, J. D., Coppen, A., Swade, C. C., and Wood, K. M. (1982): Adv. Neurol., 33:233.
9. Couch, J. R., and Hassanein, R. S. (1977): Neurology, 27:643.
10. D'Andrea, G., Toldo, M., Cananzi, A., and Ferro-Milone, F. (1984): Stroke, 15:271.
11. Deshmukh, S. V., and Meyer, J. S. (1977): Headache, 17:101.
12. Edmeads, J. (1977): Headache. 17:148.
13. Fanchamps, A. (1974): Can. J. Neurol. Sci., :189.
14. Gawel, M., Burkitt, M., and Rose, F. C. (1979): Headache, 19:323.
15. Geaney, E. R., Rutherford, M., Elliott, M., Schacter, M., and Grahame-Smith, D. G. (1983): Proceed. 1st International Headache Congress, p. 64.
16. Gelmers, H. J. (1982): Cephalagia, 2:29.
17. Glover, V., Peatfield, R., Zammit-Pace, R.-M., Littlewood, J., Gawel, M., Rose, F. C., and Sandler, M. (1981): J. Neurol. Neurosurg. Psychiat., 44:786.
18. Glover, V., Sandler, M., Grant, E., Rose, F. C., Orton, D., Wilkinson, M., and Stevens, D. (1977): Lancet, 1:391.
19. Hachinski, V. C., et al. (1978): In: Current Concepts in Migraine Research, edited by R. Greene, pp. 11-15. Raven Press, New York.
20. Hanington, E. (1979): Biomed., 30:65.
21. Hanington, E., Jones, R. J., and Amess, J. A. L. (1982): Lancet, 1:437.
22. Harvey, J. A., and Lints, C. E. (1965): Science, 148:250.
23. Hilton, B. P., and Cumings, J. N. (1971): J. Clin. Pathol., 24:250.
24. Hilton, B. P., and Cumings, J. N. (1972): J. Neurol. Neurosurg. Psychiat., 35:505.
25. Jones, R. J., Forsythe, A. M., and Amess, J. A. L. (1982): Adv. Neurol., 33:275.
26. Kalendovsky, Z., and Austin, J. H. (1975): Headache, 15:18.
27. Kangasniemi, P., Sonninen, V., and Rinne, U. K. (1972): Headache, 12:62.
28. Krivanek, J. (1977): Brain Res., 120:493.

29. Lance, J. W., and Anthony, M. (1971): Med. J. Aust., 1:242.
30. Launay, J. M., Pradalier, A., Dreux, D., and Dry, J. (1982): Cephalagia, 2:57.
31. Lindegaard, K. F., Ovrelid, L., and Sjaastad, O. (1980): Headache, 20:96.
32. Malmgren, R., Olsson, P., Tornling, G., and Unge, G. (1978): Thromb. Res., 13:1137.
33. Masel, B. E., Chesson, A. L., Alperin, J. B., Levin, H. S., and Peters, B. H. (1978): Neurology, 28:371.
34. Mathew, N. T., Hrastnik, F., and Meyer, J. (1976): Headache, 16:252.
35. Murphy, D. L., and Donnelly, C. H. (1974): In: Neuropsychopharmacology of Monoamines And Their Regulatory Enzymes, edited by E. Usdin, pp. 71–85. Raven Press, New York.
36. Muck-Seler, D., Deanovic, Z., and Dupelj, M. (1979): Headache, 19:14.
37. O'Brien, M. D. (1967): Lancet, 1:1036.
38. O'Brien, M. D. (1971): Headache, 10:139.
39. Olesen, J., Larsen, B., and Lauritzen, M. (1981): Ann. Neurol., 10:344.
40. Peatfield, R. C., and Rose, F. C. (1981): Headache, 21:140.
41. Poloni, M., Nappi, G., Arrigo, A., and Savoldi, F. (1974): Experientia, 30:640.
42. Roberts, P. J. (1973): Brain Res., 49:451.
43. Rydzewski, W., and Wachowicz, B. (1978): In: Current Concepts in Migraine Research, edited by R. Greene. Raven Press, New York.
44. Sakai, F., and Meyer, J. (1978): Headache, 18:122.
45. Sakai, F., and Meyer, J. (1979): Headache, 19:257.
46. Sandler, M., Youdim, M. B. H., and Hanington, E. (1974): Nature, 250:335.
47. Sandler, M., Youdim, M. B. H., Southgate, J., and Hanington, E. (1970): In: Background to Migraine, 3rd Migraine Symposium, edited by A. L. Cochran, pp. 103–112. William Heinemann Medical Books Ltd., London.
48. Sicuteri, F. (1971): Pharm. Res. Comm., 3:401.
49. Sicuteri, F. (1972): Headache, 12:69.
50. Sicuteri, F., Buffoni, F., Anselmi, B., and Del Bianco, D. L. (1972): Res. Clin. Stud. Headache, 3:245.
51. Sicuteri, F., Testi, A., and Anselmi, B. (1961): Int. Arch. Allergy Appl. Immun., 19:55.
52. Simard, D., and Paulson, O. B. (1973): Arch. Neurol., 29:207.
53. Skinhoj, E. (1973): Arch. Neurol., 29:95.
54. Stensrud, P., and Sjaastad, O. (1974): Headache, 14:96.
55. Thomas, V. (1982): Adv. Neurol., 33:279.
56. Wachowicz, B. (1982): Adv. Neurol., 33:243.
57. Waldenlind, E., Saaf, J., Ekbom, K., Ross, S., Wahlund, L.-O., and Wetterberg, L. (1983): Kinetics and thermolability of platelet monoamine oxidase in cluster headache and migraine. Cephalagia,

58. Welch, K. M. A., Chabi, E., Nell, J. H., Bartosk, K., Chee, A. N. C., Mathew, N. T., and Achar, V. S. (1976): Headache, 16:160.
59. Welch, K. M. A., Kite, L. D., and Keenan, P. A. (1982): In: Prostaglandins, Platelets and Salicylates: Basic and Clinical Aspects. Postgraduate Medicine, pp. 89-96.
60. Welch, K. M. A., Spira, P. J., Knowles, L., et al. (1974): Neurology, 24:705.
61. Wolff, H. G. (1962): Headache and Other Head Pain, 2nd Edition, pp. 227-301. Oxford University Press, New York.
62. Wu, K. K., and Hoak, J. C. (1974): Lancet, 2:924.

The Management of Headache, edited by F. Clifford Rose. Raven Press, New York © 1988.

VASCULAR ASPECTS OF MIGRAINE PATHOPHYSIOLOGY

Jes Olesen

Department of Neuromedicine,
Københavns amts sygehus i Gentofte,
2900 Hellerup, Denmark

REGIONAL CEREBRAL BLOOD FLOW (rCBF) DURING ATTACKS OF CLASSIC MIGRAINE

We studied four series of patients during attacks of classic migraine (2-5) where most of the important CBF abnormalities were found. rCBF was virtually always reduced during the aura phase of the attack and the reduction persisted in most patients into the headache phase. The reduced blood flow started at the posterior pole of the hemisphere and spread gradually anteriorly to a varying extent, sometimes finally involving the whole hemisphere, in other cases stopping at central sulcus or even further posteriorly. Hypoperfusion thus did not respect territories of supply of major cerebral arteries, which made it unlikely that the reduction could be due to vasospasm in such an artery. The reduction was about 35% in the focal area and sometimes even less.

Various functional tests were carried out, such as opening the eyes, listening, speaking and moving the hand. In the area of reduced blood flow, such activation procedures did not cause the usual focal increase of cerebral blood flow, whereas activation outside the focal area was normal. Finally, rCBF did not increase in the headache phase of the attack, even where patients were followed for several hours, even though others, using different techniques, found moderate increases of cerebral blood flow during and after classic migraine attacks (7). We also observed focal hyperemia in three patients preceding migrainous symptoms and hypoperfusion, but this was not observed in later series and its significance is uncertain.

Since arteriography, or the intracarotid CBF procedure itself, can trigger classic migraine attacks, it was possible to design a prospective series of studies in patients suspected of having classic migraine, where there was no positive family history, so that angiography was indicated to rule out an intracranial A-V malformation.

In these prospective studies (3,4) most of the above mentioned features were confirmed, and it was also possible to correlate closely clinical symptoms and rCBF changes. rCBF was often reduced in the very posterior aspect of the hemisphere before symptoms developed, and the reduced blood flow often persisted after all aura symptoms had disappeared. Blood flow studies were repeated at only 5-10 minute intervals, which made it possible to follow the spread of reduced blood flow more closely and to calculate the rate of spread to 2.2 mm/min. In this calculation, the involution of the cortex was not taken into account so that the actual speed of progression is probably higher. The spreading hypoperfusion did not cross the central or lateral sulcus, but appeared in the frontal lobe apparently independent of the posterior oligemia, indicating that it had spread through the insular cortex. The mode of spread and the relatively poor association in time between focal symptoms and hypoperfusion indicated that symptoms were not caused by hypoperfusion. The findings are much more compatible with a primary disorder of cerebral cortex resulting in symptoms and in hypoperfusion.

It was also possible to demonstrate normal cerebral autoregulation, i.e., constancy in cerebral blood flow during moderate blood pressure changes (3), and this occurred in the unaffected cortex as well as in the hypoperfused cortex. On the contrary, the responsiveness to changes in arterial PCO_2 was reduced. This is a very special pattern, since autoregulation is usually much more sensitive to other disturbing influences than PCO_2 reactivity.

Since attacks are induced by the intracarotid technique, it could be asked whether the findings were representative of spontaneous classic migraine attacks. We therefore studied a series of eleven patients during spontaneous attacks of classic migraine using inhalation of radioactive Xenon and single photon emission computerized tomography (SPECT) (2). In these patients, who came to the Acute Headache Clinic in Copenhagen for treatment of their usual attacks and were then asked to participate in the blood flow studies, the findings were essentially the same. The patients were studied a few hours after the onset of the attack, some still having aura symptoms, others being in the beginning of the headache phase. Eight patients displayed hypoperfusion, and three patients a normal blood flow. Reduced blood flow was located in the cortical mantle and did not affect (or only very slightly) deeper structures.

Spread of oligemia was not demonstrated at this stage of the attack, but reduced blood flow can persist for several hours after termination of aura symptoms; cerebral hyperemia was not present during the first hours of the untreated attack, or after treatment when the patients were symptom free. Comparison with studies done when patients had been free from migraine for at least a week showed no difference from normal controls.

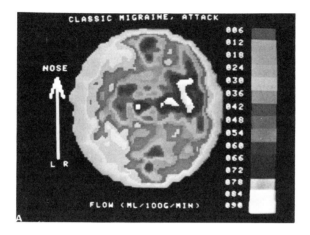

FIG. 1. Tomographic recording of regional cerebral blood flow during a classic migraine attack. On the scale to the right blood flow values in ml/100 g/min are translated into shades of gray. The rim around the picture is outside of the brain. On the right side the brain cortex is dark. On the left side the same area is light gray, indicating a much reduced cerebral blood flow in virtually all of the left hemispheric cortex.

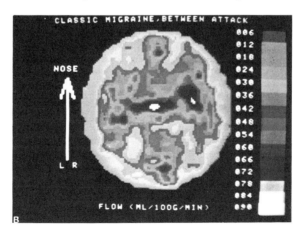

FIG. 2. Same patient as FIG. 1., now outside of a migraine attack. Note a fairly good symmetry in the picture and no evidence of hypoperfusion. This cut is a little deeper than FIG. 1., which is why the flow in the right hemisphere looks slightly different.

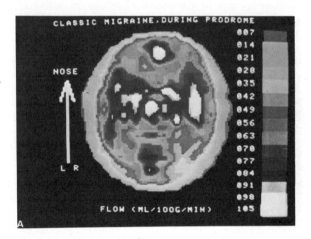

FIG. 3.   Blood flow map during prodromes of classic migraine with left-sided homonymous visual disturbances.   The left occipital region is normal, but regional cerebral blood flow is reduced in the right occipital region corresponding to the symptoms.

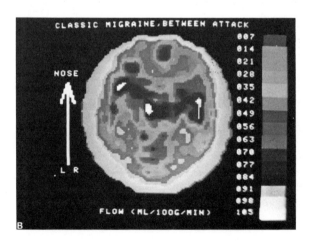

FIG. 4.   Same patient as FIG. 3., now outside of attack and with a completely normal blood flow map.

CEREBRAL BLOOD FLOW STUDIES DURING ATTACKS OF COMMON MIGRAINE

Twelve patients with spontaneous attacks of common migraine attending the Acute Headache Clinic in Copenhagen for treatment of their attacks (2) were also studied. Measurements taken from 7 to 20 hours after the onset of the attack showed no significant alterations of focal or global cerebral blood flow.

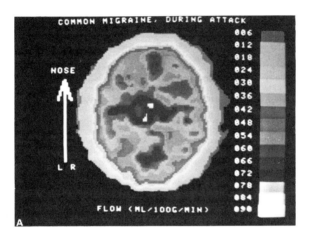

FIG. 5.   Patient studied during a common migraine attack.   The blood   flow   map   is   completely   symmetric   with   no   focal abnormalities.

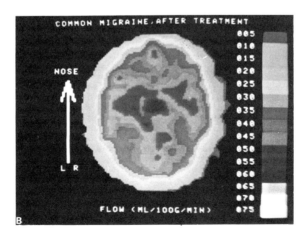

FIG. 6.   Same patient as FIG. 5., now after treatment.   The blood   flow   map   is   still   symmetric   and   not   significantly different from the study during the attack.

Although these patients were studied later than the patients with classic migraine, reduced blood flow would be expected in some if the pathological process was the same as in classic migraine.

To study whether the common migraine attacks had been initiated by reduced cerebral blood flow, we provoked attacks by red wine (6). Three patients were studied twice using different techniques, i.e., inhalation of radioactive Xenon with external stationary detectors or with tomography. One patient was studied by intracarotid injection of 133-Xenon when she developed a spontaneous common migraine attack. Measurements taken in these patients before and after provocation and repeated until patients were into the fully developed common migraine attack showed no changes, either of cerebral hypoperfusion or hyperperfusion.

These results strongly indicate that common migraine is not associated with the blood flow changes typical of classic migraine, and the two types of migraine should therefore always be studied independently.

CLASSIC MIGRAINE AND THE SPREADING DEPRESSION OF LEAO

Leao's spreading depression (SD) is a response that can be elicited in the cerebral cortex by a variety of stimuli. Pathophysiologically, intensive bursts of action potentials followed by depolarization of neurons and glial cells and marked electrolyte changes with equilibration of potassium and sodium across the cellular membrane is seen. This phenomenon spreads gradually across the cortex at a rate of 3 mm/min. Immediately after depolarization, restoration of normal electrolyte gradients starts. This requires energy and focal cerebral glucose consumption increases about 200% (8), and there is also increased lactic acid production and pH shifts. The process is associated with marked slow tissue potentials changes and, following the wave of SD, normal EEG activity is depressed for 5-10 minutes. The SD is thus comparable to a wave which slowly moves across the cerebral cortex. The wave itself is only 2-3 mm wide and, within the wave, rCBF is markedly increased in parallel with metabolism. In the wake of SD, cerebral blood flow is depressed for long periods (1) and the regulation of cerebral blood flow remains impaired. Autoregulation is normal, but responsiveness to PCO_2-changes is reduced.

SD is most easily elicited in rodents and other small animals, probably because of their high neurone density. The elicitation can be caused by local application of concentrated potassium, focal injuries, other mechanical stimulation and microinjections of homologous blood. The cortex can be sensitized to elicitation of SD by flushing with high potassium solutions, depolarizing amino acids, agents which block the sodium pump and systemic administration of metrazole.

RELATION BETWEEN BLOOD FLOW CHANGES IN MIGRAINE
AND THE SPREADING DEPRESSION OF LEAO

A number of characteristic features of rCBF changes during classic migraine attacks and after SD are the same, especially the spread of oligemia. The onset of hypoperfusion (and perhaps SD) can be explained by the high neurone density in the visual cortex. The rate of spread of cerebral oligemia and of SD is approximately the same. In most focal brain lesions, such as tumors, stroke, trauma, etc., cerebral autoregulation is impaired, but PCO_2 reactivity is often preserved. The opposite is seen during classic migraine attacks as well as in animals after a wave of SD. The confinement of changes to the cerebral cortical mantle during classic migraine attacks and after SD is a rather specific feature. The hyperemic zone seen in animals during SD may not be seen in the human because it is only 2-3 mm wide and moves, which makes it extremely hard and perhaps impossible to detect with current CBF techniques in man. It is an open question whether the initial focal hyperemia observed in three patients in our first series could represent such a hyperemic wave of SD.

At present there are so many parallels between the animal experimental phenomenon of SD of Leao, and observations during classic migraine attacks, that the relationship between the two conditions should be studied further. It would indeed be a great step forward if an animal experimental model of classic migraine could be established.

SUMMARY

Regional cerebral blood flow (rCBF) is usually depressed during the aura phase of classic migraine and remains so into the headache phase. The reduction measured ranges from 10% - 40%, but may in reality be greater. It has a typical developmental pattern starting at the posterior pole of the hemisphere and progressing anteriorly. In some patients it finally involves the whole hemisphere, but in most it stops before. The rate of progression is 2-3 mm per minute. In the hypoperfused area, functional activation, e.g., by hand movement, does not result in the usual focal blood flow increase. The response to increased arterial PCO_2 is reduced, but regulation to changes in blood pressure is normal. We have not observed increased blood flow in the pain phase of classic migraine attacks. In common migraine no abnormalities in any phase of the attacks were observed, and we believe that common migraine despite its similarities with classic migraine should be regarded as a pathophysiologically separate entity. The animal experimental model of spreading depression of cortical electrical activity, also called spreading depression of Leao, resembles in many ways the rCBF abnormalities observed in classic migraine. It is so far the best bid for an animal experimental model of migraine.

Acknowledgement:

   This chapter is a summary of a series of studies done in collaboration with Doctors Martin Lauritzen, Anker Jon Hansen, Tom Skyhøj Olsen, Peer Tfelt-Hansen, Leif Henriksen, and Bo Larsen. The role of the other investigators is apparent from the list of references.

REFERENCES

1. Lauritzen, M., Balslev Jørgensen, M., Diemer, N. H., Gjedde, A., and Hansen, A. J. (1982): Ann. Neurol., 12:469.
2. Lauritzen, M., and Olesen, J. (1984): Brain, 104:447.
3. Lauritzen, M., Skyhøj Olsen, T., Lassen, N. A., and Paulson, O. B. (1983): Ann. Neurol., 14:569.
4. Lauritzen, M., Skyhøj Olsen, T., Lassen, N. A., and Paulson, O. B. (1983): Ann. Neurol., 16:463.
5. Olesen, J., Larsen, B., and Lauritzen, M. (1981): Ann. Neurol., 9:344.
6. Olesen, J., Tfelt-Hansen, P., Henriksen, L., and Larsen, B. (1981): Lancet, 2:438.
7. Sakai, F., and Meyer, J. S. (1978): Headache, 18:122.
8. Shinohara, M., Dollinger, B., Brown, G., Rapoport, S., and Sokoloff, L. (1979): Science, 203:188.

The Management of Headache,
by F. Clifford Rose. Raven Pres.
New York © 1988.

THE BIOCHEMISTRY OF MIGRAINE

George W. Bruyn, MD DSc

Chairman, Department of Neurology, Academic Hospital,
State University, Leiden, The Netherlands

and

M. D. Ferrari

Department of Neurology, Academic Hospital,
State University, Leiden, The Netherlands

Although a considerable quantity of biochemical research has been going on in recent years (17,18), a specific (not to say pathognomonic) chemical parameter of the migraine attack has still eluded identification. As long as such a parameter remains unknown, unequivocal diagnosis and ultimately successful treatment will remain utopian rather than realistic.

The present state of affairs, characterized by the failure of a breakthrough to materialize, calls for reconsideration of those factors to which this failure can be attributed. The first question to arise, of course, is what available evidence would warrant the presumption that migraine is a disease entity based upon a single chemical causative agent or process. The empirical fact that migraine attacks are precipitated by a wide range of disparate factors, stress grantedly being the most common, in apparently genetically predisposed individuals, only the attack per se showing an exquisitely stereotyped sequence of events, such as prodromes, aura, pain, vegetative dysfunction, sleep (18), makes it fairly likely that migraine is a syndrome rather than a nosological disease-entity. Indeed, some workers do not even accept the monotonous cascade-like sequence of symptoms of the migraine attack as a characteristic feature (88), suggesting instead a single central factor producing different symptoms due to impact at different sites.

The next query may well be whether common and classic migraine are in essence identical. There is some evidence to the contrary: serotonin-induced platelet aggregability is increased in classic (100) but not in common migraine, and inversely, circulating immune complexes and complement activation appear to manifest in common but not in classic migraine (71). Platelet 5HT compartmentation differs in both conditions (75). Prolactin plasma levels react normally (decrease) in common migraineurs in response to L–Dopa. On the contrary, in classical migraine prolactin plasma levels increase (101).

The old clinical distinction between white and red migraineurs found a recent pendant in a study demonstrating two groups, the majority showing serotoninergic mechanisms to predominate over catecholaminergic systems, and a minority in which the opposite obtained (67). The most obvious question, viz. if migraine in women has a differential biochemical (e.g. hormonal) causation from that in men, before lumping them together in a study, as if their common identity is a priori self-evident, is still an open question. Last but not least comes the consideration that even in a study of homogeneous and sufficiently large patient material (i.e. at least 20 patients), carefully selected for the factors of age, sex, diagnosis, identical times of biological fluid specimen-sampling, before, during, after the attack and in the attack-free interval, identical, pre-, per-, post-trial dietary regimen, and work-up of an optimal control series, in short, with impecable methodology, many studies differ in techniques of biochemical assay, making comparison difficult if not altogether impossible.

A synopsis of biochemical findings that grosso modo seem to have been reasonably established can perhaps be best presented in the Tables 1–4.

TABLE 1.

PLASMA

During the Attack	Between Attacks
* Na↓	↑
* DA-beta-H↑	?
* cAMP ↑	?
* FFA linoleic	?
* FFA oleic ↑	?
* FFA palmitic	?
Free Tryptophan↑	?
* 5-HT↓	?
* Beta-endorphin ↓	?
* Beta-TG ↑	?
* PF4	?
* Estradiol↑	↓
Aldosterone↑	↓?
Renin ↑	↓
Cortisol: aberrant circadian pattern	
Insulin response to glucose	↓

The Management of Headache, edited by F. Clifford Rose. Raven Press, New York © 1988.

TABLE 2.

PLATELETS

During the Attack	Between Attacks
Adhesiveness ⎫ ↓	↑
Aggregability ⎭	
MAO-B (males) ↓	↓ (males)
PSP-T↓(dietary M.)	↓(dietary M.)
Total nucleotides↑	?
ADP ↑	
Taurine↑	?
5-HT ⎫	
Beta-TG ⎬ ↓	
PF4 ⎭	
5-HT-reuptake ↓	↓
Polyunsat. FFA ⎫	
Arachidonic A ⎭	
(in phospholipids↑)	

TABLE 3.

CEREBROSPINAL FLUID

* Lactate   ↑
* GABA   ↑
* cAMP   ↑
* TRY   ↑
* HVA   ↑
* Proteases   ↑
* Beta-endorph.   ↓
  (met-enkeph.)

TABLE 4.

URINE

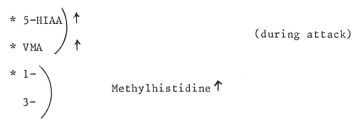

* 5-HIAA ⎫ ↑
        ⎬   (during attack)
* VMA ⎭ ↑

* 1- ⎫
     ⎬ Methylhistidine ↑
  3- ⎭

This apparently heterogeneous set of changes can be construed into a fairly coherent flow-chart (98) represented in Figure 1.

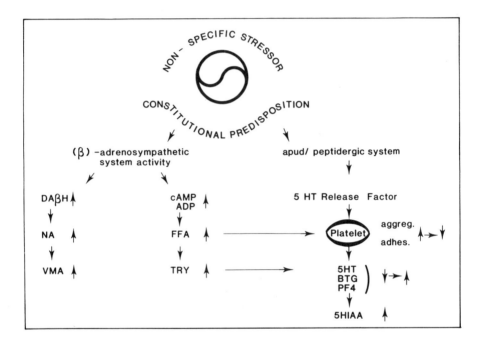

This flow-chart does not, of course, account for all the pharmacological and biochemical observations made over the last few decades, nor does it in any definite measure "explain" the migraine attack, but it puts a number of findings arrived at by systemic research in rational sequence.

The biochemical and neuropharmacological research in migraine today proceeds along a number of main avenues:

The Platelet/Serotonin Theory

Kimball and Goodman (60), and later Sicuteri (85,86) found that migraine headache was markedly relieved by intravenous administration of 5-hydroxytryptamine (5-HT) or its precursor 5-hydroxytryptophan (5-HTP). Dalessio (25) proposed that the efficacy of methysergide in migraine was due to its 5-HT inhibitory action. Sicuteri, Testi and Anselmi (93) noted markedly increased urinary excretion of the main metabolite of

5-HT, 5-hydroxyindoleacetic acid (5-HIAA), during the migraine attack. Although Southren and Christoff (97) found normal CSF 5-HT values during the migraine attack, and Curzon et al. (24) failed to detect significant urinary 5-HIAA variations in migraine, subsequent work (6,23,52,53,59,96) confirmed that urinary 5-HIAA and vanyl mandelic acid (VMA) increased during the first twelve hours of the attack and that plasma 5-HT as well as noradrenaline (NA) (34) fall shortly before the attack in most subjects. These findings were again confirmed by Anthony (4,5,6,) in a series of carefully executed experiments in which an increase of long-chain fatty acids (palmitic, oleic, and linoleic) was revealed, with an increase in platelet nucleotides, adenosine diphosphate (ADP) being greater than adenosine triphosphate (ATP), confirmed by Rydzewski (83), free 5-HT being excreted in the urine.

In the course of the seventies, it was shown (43,84,85) that platelet monoamine oxidase (MAO) B-type (of which the substrates are tyramine, dopamine, and 2-phenylethylamine) is transiently decreased, be it only in male migraineurs (42). Although this apparently contradicts the finding that MAO inhibitors exert beneficial effects in migraine (5), it would seem to tie in with the observation that tyramine administration provokes migraine attacks in some diet-sensitive migraineurs. However, platelet MAO activity is lower still in cluster headache (and therefore not migraine specific), and not correlated with platelet size or migraine (81).

Anthony, Hinterberger and Lance (5) postulated the appearance in plasma of a factor releasing 5-HT from platelets, a postulate that has been confirmed (27,31,77,78). This serotonin-releasing factor (SRF) activating the platelet is as yet unidentified, though its molecular weight appears to be between 5 and 10 KD (Anthony, personal communication, 1984). Recently Launay and Pradalier (65) made it plausible that the SRF also inhibits 5-HT reuptake during an attack. Furthermore, during common migraine attacks, they were able to show a decrease in the platelet content of other dense body constituents viz catecholamines, together with a rise in the plasma levels. They suggested that the SRF releases 5-HT via dense body release. Platelet activation is confirmed by its release of beta-thromboglobulin (38) and PF4 (26) and by the increased aggregability of platelets before the attacks (22,58), and their reduced aggregability afterward.

It seems, therefore, reasonably well established that the indolamine 5-HT is involved, as well as the catecholamine NA (both showing a a pre- and per-attack decrease), that MAO activity is decreased, and that there must be something wrong with the platelet because: 1) 5-HT releasing factor is effective only with platelets from migraineurs and not with those from healthy people (77,78); 2) 5-HT uptake by platelets in migraineurs is deranged (21,40,72,82), although found normal by others showing an unduly large granule storage compartment in the intervals (75); 3) imipramine binding (on a site associated with active 5-HT uptake) is significantly reduced even between attacks in classic migraine; and 4) because of changed platelet nucleotides (48) and FFA profiles (80) although others found normal platelet lipid composition (16).   Also, in migraineurs platelets show an increased tendency to aggregate (22,49), and they seem to contain more methionine-enkephalin which is thought to be stored subcellularly in the same organelles as 5-HT (30,76).   Interestingly, the methionine-enkephalin levels do not change during a migraine episode as opposed to those of 5-HT (76).

Confirmation has come recently from various sources: Platelets by active uptake contain roughly 450 times more of the amino acid taurine than plasma (1), which increases even more during the migraine attack (29).   Also, platelets of patients with dietary migraine (though not those with non-dietary migraine) show reduced levels of the phenol-inactivating (P-) form of phenolsulphotransferase (70).   The PST-P-defect was approached by Hanington et al. (47), who noticed that dietary migraineurs upon tyramine-loading excrete significantly less free and O-sulphate-conjugated tyramine and less normetanephrine than do controls, a finding confirmed by Leupreux and Bonnet, but subsequently cast into doubt by others (61).   Intriguingly, Parkinson patients usually excrete vastly more conjugated tyramine than do normal persons, and start to excrete significantly less of it as soon as they are put upon L-Dopa therapy (14); yet they hardly ever complain of migraine.

The platelet is often used as a model for monoaminergic neurons: they take up, store, transport and release 5-HT, NA, DA and other amines, they are depleted from these amines by such well-known neuroleptic agents as reserpine, tetrabenazine and fenfluramine, as well as by tricyclic anti-depressants; they contain the enzymes MAO-A and -B, and neuron-specific enolase (73).   Little wonder then that, in view of the findings of pivotal platelet behavior in migraine, the disorder was considered to be a platelet disease (49).

The concept of migraine as a platelet disorder (thrombocytopathy) certainly offers the charm of simplicity, but whether it is true is another matter: certain changes of both physiological and biochemical nature occur before the migraineur's deviant platelet gets actively involved, such as the production of a platelet SRF.

The concept does, however, have the virtue of reconciling the neurogenic and humoral aspects of migraine.   The non-specificity of triggers (denying a single causative factor) filtered by the CNS, and the stereotyped course of the attack once unleashed (underlining the probability of a "final common path"), seem to be admirably explained by the platelet theory.

The Neurotransmitter Dysfunction Theory
(Opioid Hypofunction + Dopamine Hyperfunction)

This theory combines various clinical, biochemical and pharmacological observations into one framework, namely that of failure of the central opioid system in migraine. As a consequence, many other systems are deranged and produce simultaneously the different symptoms of the migraine attack (88),

This thesis implies that the dysfunctioning central opioid system modulates other systems containing neurotransmitters, such as dopamine, noradrenaline, acetylcholine, serotonin and substance P. The theory was prompted by the clinical observation of the remarkable resemblance between the migraine attack and the morphine withdrawal syndrome, both consisting of the triad: apathy (anhedonia), dysautonomia, and lowering of the pain threshold (hypernociception); by analogy, it is also called the "endorphin abstinence syndrome" (86). Histochemical and neurophysiological data (46,92) indicate that enkephalins, like the endorphins belonging to the group of opioids, show the highest concentration in the striatum, peri-aqueductal gray, brainstem, and spinal substantia gelatinosa. Here, they appear to be contained in short interneurons with inhibitory action on neurotransmitter release through mainly presynaptically located receptors. It has been shown that some opiate peptides and amines may indeed coexist within the same neurons.

One of the best known examples of interaction between an opioid system and neurotransmission concerns pain perception: From the nucleus raphe magnus, serotoninergic fibers descend through the dorsal longitudinal funiculus. Via enkephalinergic interneurons, they inhibit presynaptically the substance P containing neurons which subserve "pain-transmission" to the spinothalamic tract (10,86). Failure of the enkephalinergic system will result in increased pain perception. Besides pain modulation, the opioid system is also involved in modulating "hedonia", i.e. the sense of well-being, and the autonomic nervous system. Here, the opioid system inhibits presynaptically the release of dopamine and noradrenaline from neuron terminals. The theory holds that, as a result of dysfunction of this inhibiting system, neurotransmitters leak continuously from the terminals so that the organism reaches an "empty neuron" state, which produces postsynaptic receptor hypersensitivity, both dopaminergic and noradrenergic (88).

Since the concept was construed, numerous clinical, biochemical and pharmacological arguments have been gathered in its support. The most important observations are:

1) the very poor, and promptly tachyphylactic, analgesia from morphine and heroin in migraine pain, suggesting a mu-receptor deficiency (88);

2) the administration of intravenous pentazocine (an agonist of sigma-opiate receptors) provokes visual and body image distortions in migraineurs. Naloxone, a specific opiate

antagonist, prevents or reverts these pentazocine-induced disorders of percpetion (91);

3) Naloxone injected at the onset of the scotoma interrupts the visual phenomena in the majority of classic migraineurs. When it does, it also reduces the headache intensity and the duration of the pain. Naloxone proves ineffective in common migraine (91);

4) Naloxone promptly reversed the neurological deficits accompanying the attacks in two cases of non-familial hemiplegic migraine without influencing the pain (20);

5) Both CSF enkephalin and plasma beta-endorphin (BEP) levels were decreased in migraine attacks, whereas in migraine-free periods both were normal (3,8). In addition, CSF enkephalin levels in cluster headache and plasma BEP in chronic headache sufferers were also decreased. Bach et al. (7), however, were not able to confirm the plasma BEP level drop during an attack, even noting the slight rise instead, a discrepancy attributed to a different radio-immuno-assay (RIA) method with less cross-reaction against beta-lipoprotein. Gawel et al. (39) succeeded in showing plasma BEP decrease of minus 200-300% in classical, but not in common migraine. Furthermore, during a recent Migraine Symposium, Sicuteri et al. (92) presented new data on the plasma levels of enkephalinase (EKA), an enkephalin degrading enzyme. It was shown that in common migraine sufferers during headache-free periods, EKA levels were only 50% of those in healthy controls, and about normal during an attack. In chronic daily headache sufferers, plasma EKA levels were significantly higher than controls, while they were normal in CSF (Sicuteri, personal communication, 1985);

6) tachyphylaxis for 5-HT or tyramine induced dorsal hand vein spasm normally occurs in non-headache sufferers but there is an absence or even inversion in migraineurs and addicts. In addicts, as opposed to migraine patients, morphine will reverse this reaction resulting in tachyphylaxis (89);

7) no naloxone induced increase of luteinizing hormone (LH) plasma levels in late (and mid) luteal phase of menstrually related (and unrelated) migraine (Nappi et al., 1984, in press).

The following observations support the postulated dopaminergic receptor hypersensitivity:

1) clinical observations suggest an association between migraine and diseases or conditions with supposed dopamine hyperfunction, such as chorea (19) and Tourette's disease (9). The first source reviewed nine cases of migraine-attack-bound involuntary movements; the second source signalled a higher than expected rate in children for coexistence of Tourette's disease and migraine (26%). In addition, some clinical neurologists consider that migraine and Parkinson's disease (dopamine hypofunction) are mutually exclusive. In this context, it seems appropriate to recall the decreasing effect of opiates on striatal dopamine release, as well as the observed reduction of striatal metenkephalin in Huntington's chorea, a disease in which dopamine hyperfunction seems to be well established (46);

2) In syncopal or basilar artery migraine, patients sometimes lose consciousness during an attack. During attack-free periods migraineurs, especially those with this type of migraine, react more seriously to an oral dose of 2.5 mg bromocriptine (a dopamine D2-receptor agonist) when standing up, after having been lying in a supine position for one hour (33,90,92). They also faint more frequently than do non-migraineurs and this was always associated with a significantly greater fall in systolic and diastolic blood pressure without associated compensatory tachycardia. Domperidone (10 mg I.M.), a selective dopamine D2-receptor antagonist which poorly crosses the blood-brain-barrier (BBB), prevented or counteracted this orthostatic hypotensive effect of bromocriptine, if administered shortly before or three hours after. Interestingly, the hypotensive action of bromocriptine in migraine patients was not accompanied by the normally occurring compensatory physiological increase in sympathetic activity in view of the absence of any change in dopamine-beta-hydroxylase, nor, clinically, with an associated compensatory tachycardia. This can be interpreted as a purely central effect on the dopamine-dependent cells in blood pressure regulating centers outside the BBB (104), or as an exhaustion of the peripheral sympathetic system according to the "empty neuron" hypothesis;

3) According to Sicuteri (92), apomorphine (a dopamine D2-receptor agonist) is the only known drug to reproduce migraine-like phenomena in migraine sufferers, but not in non-headache sufferers in the same low doses. Repetition of the same dose induces tolerance with gradual disappearance of the apomorphine-evoked phenomena (headache, nausea, vomiting, shivering, orthostatic hypotension). Haloperidol, a dopamine-receptor-antagonist which crosses the BBB, prevents all these phenomena. Domperidone prevents only those phenomena presumably provoked in centers located outside the BBB, but not the centrally originated pain;

4) In patients with complete migraine who can predict an impending attack on the basis of certain premonitory signs, an oral dose of 40 mg domperidone (taken at least six but preferably twelve hours before appearance of the headache) prevented 63% of the imminent attacks (13). Placebo did so in only 5% (2,102). If domperidone was taken less than six hours before the onset of the headache, its effect was significantly less;

5) Bes et al (11,12,41) demonstrated a dopaminergic hypersensitivity at the level of the cerebral arterioles in migraineurs and suggested its use as a diagnostic test. In ten non-cephalalgic control subjects, administration of 0.2 mg/kg IV piribedil, a dopaminergic agonist which crosses the BBB and has less peripheral effects than apomorphine, produces a 22% increase in cerebral blood flow (CBF), whereas a dose of 0.1 mg/kg did not produce any significant CBF increase. Instead, in 20 common migraine patients in migraine-free periods, the same low doses (0.1 mg/kg) produced 18% (10%-39%) CBF increase in 18

subjects. It also caused (in contradistinction to controls) peripheral side-effects like nausea, vomiting, and a mean arterial blood pressure drop of 32%. Domperidone (20 mg per os) given in advance prevented the peripheral side-effects, but not the CBF change.

6) It has been demonstrated in an animal model that, after chronic administration, estrogen withdrawal was followed by hypersensitivity to dopamine agonists, presumably caused by an increase in the number of dopamine receptors (44). An important role has been attributed to estrogen withdrawal in menstrual migraine (94);

7) Recent data concerning pain modulation attribute a role to the so-called diencephalospinal dopaminergic system next to the well established influence of the descending serotoninergic fibers originating from the nucleus raphe magnus (56).

In summary, it can be concluded that the dopaminergic system must play some part in the pathogenesis of the migraine attack, at least in the very beginning, since in spontaneous attacks domperidone has an effect only if administered at least 6-12 hours before the headache starts.

The observation that domperidone is effective in preventing attacks implies that other neurotransmitters, such as histamine, serotonin, and other catecholamines are less important during the first part of the attack since, in the dose used, the receptor binding profile of domperidone includes only dopaminergic D2 (= not-cAMP mediated) receptors (68).

One might argue that some drugs effective in migraine prophylaxis, such as clonidine and propranolol, do not share this D2-antagonistic property (68).

There is a discrepancy between the ability of domperidone to prevent the headache in spontaneous attacks but not the pain or CBF changes in drug-induced attacks, in contradistinction to centrally-acting dopamine antagonists. Since domperidone is unable to cross the intact BBB, the hypothesis of a (temporary morphological or functional) defective BBB during a migraine attack could be more valid than has been appreciated up to now (51). In this respect, it would be interesting to know whether domperidone is also able to counteract the pathognomonic CBF changes during and after an attack.

Finally, if the migraineur is characterized by a dopaminergic-hyperresponsive state and the attack is due to its derangement, not all dopamine systems are involved because the serum prolactin level (which is mainly regulated by D2 receptors inside the pituitary gland) does not show a significant change during an attack (103). Also, in common migraine attacks, L-Dopa infusions which normally would suppress prolactin secretion in the normal person do not produce an (expectedly exaggerated) decrease of the serum level (101). Interestingly, in complicated migraine attacks there was even an increase in the serum level.

The Propagating Negative Wave Theory

In the last few years a number of Scandinavian workers, notably Olesen and Lauritzen (79) have made a number of observations on cortical blood flow with the aid of the 133Xe-method during the migraine attack that have fundamentally changed the concepts on the pathogenesis of migraine. The traditional vasomotor theory of Wolff, essentially suggesting that vasoconstriction, vasodilatation and vascular wall edema are the pathophysiological events underlying the aura and headache stages of the attack, has been laid to rest as one of medicine's past errors. Modern evidence indicates a neurogenic rather than a vascular or humoral origin.

The Scandinavian group (see previous chapter) established that the cortical blood flow diminishes during the classic migraine attack. The hypoperfusion invariably started in the occipital lobe and spread rostrally with a speed of $\pm$ 2mm/min, disrespecting arterial supply territories. The reduction in cortical blood flow averaged 36% (15%-60%). Cortical perfusion normally is 80-105 ml. $100 \text{ gr.}^{-1} \text{ min}^{-1}$. The cerebral tolerance limit for ischemia ranges between 20 and 25 ml. $100^{-1} \text{ min}^{-1}$, with cortical electrical activity rapidly declining between 18 and 12 ml. $100^{-1} \text{ gr. min}^{-1}$ (99). The hypoperfusion preceded the aura phase or started during it, and often persisted long after the neurological symptoms had disappeared. Gulliksen and Enevoldsen (1984) noted hyperemia lasting up to 24 hours after the hypoperfusion seen during the attack. At the same time there was an impaired CO_2-response, but normal autoregulation. These changes were noted to occur nearly invariably in classic migraine, never (with one exception) in common migraine, and were once seen in a patient without migraine. The headache invariably developed when cortical hypoperfusion was still present, and is long gone when hyperperfusion is still seen.

The conclusions to be derived from these data are clear:

1) common and classic migraine differ not only clinically but also physiopathologically;

2) vasoconstriction is not the cause of neurological symptoms during the aura, in view of the limited magnitude of hypoperfusion, the temporal dysjunction between headache and CBF changes, and the absence of any relationship with arterial territories; and

3) headache is not due to intracranial vasodilatation.

Indeed, there seems no causal relationship between cortical hypoperfusion, headache and neurological deficit at all. This suggests that any future research in migraine, in which patients with the common and classic type are lumped together, should be automatically disqualified.

The slow spread of cortical hypoperfusion appears to underline earlier propositions that migrainous neurological symptoms might well be due to Leao's spreading depression (SD) of EEG activity. In the animal there is the same lack of relationship between SD and neural symptoms.

The phenomenon of SD consists of an excitation wave followed by extinction of activity, spreading at a rate of 2-3 mm/min. across the cortex; elicited by sharp or electric trauma or even mere exposure of the cortex, or application of solutions of K^+, glutamate, aspartate, or blockers of the Na-K-pump. A burst of intense firing lasting a few seconds is followed within 30 sec. by loss of action potentials for 10-15 min., during which a surface positive/negative/positive wave complex of 1-2/15-30/1-2 mV taking 3-6 min. passes by. During this wave, evoked responses cannot be obtained. The initial firing burst is associated by a 250% CBF increase lasting 1-2 min. and followed by a 25% reduction in CBF lasting one hour. This is not due to a reduced cerebral energy metabolism in view of a normal glucose consumption (66). During the SD normal neuronal activity is disrupted. The astrocytes swell, as well as the dendrites in the superficial cortex layers, and the interstitial space of the brain, being as it is the smallest of all organs, is decreased by half. Osler, with piercing insight, characterized migraine as "Hives of the brain", i.e. cerebral urticaria. This pathophysiological process involves only the superficial cortex layers and, because of its spread across the cortex at a rate of 2-3 mm/min., is eminently suited to be put on one line with such aura symptoms as the scintillating scotoma, cheirooral paresthesias, etc.

Thanks to the introduction of ion-specific micropipettes, considerable ion-changes were noted to occur during SD:

$(K^+)_e$ rises from 3 mMol $\longrightarrow$ 20 (7 to 20-fold)

$(Na^+)_e$ falls from 150 mMol $\longrightarrow$ 55 (2 to 3-fold)

$(Cl^-)_e$ falls from 130 mMol $\longrightarrow$ 79 (2 fold)

$(Ca^{++})_e$ falls from 1.3 mMol $\longrightarrow$ 0.1 (10 to 13-fold), with consequent neuronoglial depolarization and impossibility for both neurons and glia to repolarize. The restoration of the normal situation has to be carried out and requires energy: the cortical metabolic rate and glucose consumption increase 2-fold, cortical pO_2, lactate, NADH, and glycogen fall, and a CO_2-reactivity decrease is noted. The vasomotor changes are secondary to the primary neuronal changes. (For summary, see Table 5).

Gardner-Medwin (35,36,37) stressed that the astrocyte population is the cell-system par excellence to redistribute (K^+) over large neuronal distances. It is especially in man and in the occipital lobes that the ratio neuron/astrocyte is low, i.e., there is a relative shortage of glia to cope with released K^+. The glial cells form a spatial buffer, that accounts for 80% of cortical K^+-flux, and controls $(K^+)_e$ at $\pm$ 3 mMol, well under the ceiling of 12 mMol.

If for some cause or other the $(K^+)_e$ rises beyond the glial ability to cope with the uptake and redistribution of the K^+-ion over dendritic distances which are 1,000 to 10,000 times as large as the intercellular distance, the conditions are met for SD to arise. It is the glial failure that ignites the neuronal dysfunction.

TABLE 5

	SPREADING DEPRESSION	CLASSIC MIGRAINE
	DIFFERENCES	
species	lower mammals	man
site	superf.layers lissencephalic cortex cerebellum hippocampus striatum	convoluted cortex?
neuronal/glia ratio	high	low
origin	pathological physicochemical stimulus	? ("spontaneous")
features	spreading DC negat. wave, 1-2 min.	?
	250%↑ CoBF, 1-2 min.	possible
	hypoperfusion (-25%), 1 hr.	4-5 hrs.
	refractory period 1-15 min.	hours
	cortical pO_2 ↓	?
	creat.phosphate ↓	?
	phosphate ↑	?
	Co metab. rate O_2 ↑	?
	Co metab. rate glucose ↑	?
	lactic acid ↑ , cAMP ↑	↑
	GABA ↑	
	HCO_3^- ↑	
	NADH → NAD 25% ↓	?
	$[K^+]e$ 3 mMol → > 20 mMol	
	$[Na^+]e$ 150 mMol → 55 mMol	
	$[Cl^-]e$ 130 mMol → 70 mMol	) ?
	$[Ca^{2+}]e$ 1.3 mMol → 0.1 mMol	
	swelling dendrites, vol.interst. space 50%↓	
blocked by	high CO_2-inhalation	±
	cocaine, Mg, Mn, CO	?
	SIMILARITIES	
not blocked by	anaesthesia, anoxia, TTX	—
VER	↓	↓
SSEP	↓	↓ ?
art.supplyterrit.	no barrier	no barrier
anat. boundaries	barrier	?

Precisely here, humoral, vascular, and neurogenic domains intermingle. Merit is due to Gardner-Medwin (35,36) for having provided a scientific basis for the approximation between SD and migraine, which up to the appearance of his papers had never left the speculative domain. These electrolyte shifts produce considerable pH changes in the tissue compartments (cellular, interstitial); within this context the marked beneficial prophylactic and therapeutic effects of acetazolamide, a carbonic anhydrase-inhibitor, on scintillating scotoma become understandable (74).

If SD and the migraine attack indeed can be compared as largely identical pathophysiological processes, what causes can be conceived for such an event?

1) A period of locally intense neuronal firing due to overstimulation, e.g. by strong glittering lights (striate cortex);

2) high neuron/glia ratio (as normally is present in striate cortex; neurons fall out with age, as does migraine);

3) exertion, during which systemic blood pressure rises considerably, and, with it, the hydrostatic capillary pressure. If the latter rises above $\pm$ 40 mm Hg, the net filtration pressure, which drives out plasma-solutes from the arterial capillary lumen, increases 70-fold (from 0.3 to $\pm$ 20 mg Hg), producing interstitial space edema as a consequence. This is what may happen in runner's, or weight lifter's, or coital migraine, in short exertional migraine;

4) local trauma (concussion or contusion) with break-down of the BBB, and leakage of serous fluid into the interstitial space;

5) lowering of the plasma colloid osmotic pressure from 28 to 10 mm Hg, with the same consequence;

6) local lesions (angiitis, angtioma) with BBB breakdown, and identical results;

7) impairment of noradrenergic locus ceruleus function, with subsequent unilateral neurogenic impairment of BBB and leakage of serum into the interstitial gel (50). In this context it should be recalled that Sicuteri and Fanciullacci (1979) demonstrated the presence of sympathetic nervous system deficiency with denervation hypersensitivity in migraineurs. The state of insufficiency of the noradrenergic nervous system, and its lability (34), combined with parasympathetic hyperfunction has recently been proven to exist between attacks (45,62), thereby confirming the Italian, and early American, findings (63). The pre-attack alpha-noradrenergic activity burst, indicating lability of the ortho/para-sympathetic system has been reappraised in a wider context (57);

8) Speculatively, the appearance of peptide precursors or a serotonin-releasing factor and platelet dysfunction may impair the normal interplay between platelet and endothelium.

Why is the BBB and leakage of serous fluid into the interstitial space of the brain so important?

A short digression will clarify this (Figure 2).

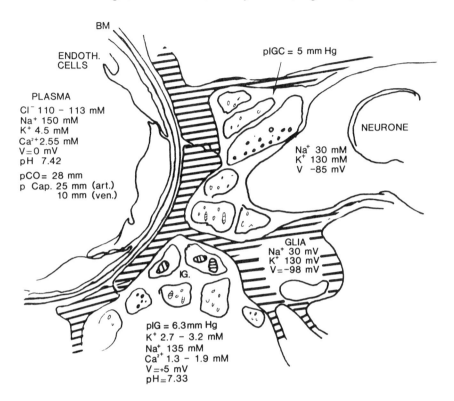

The exchange of fluid (and solutes) between the capillary lumen and the CNS tissue is controlled by four pressure forces:

i)   Colloid osmotic pressure of the blood drawing tissue fluid into the capillary lumen (pCO = 28 mm Hg)

ii) Hydrostatic blood pressure in the capillary, driving fluid from the capillary into the tissue (Pa Cap = 25 p_v cap = 10 mm Hg)

iii) Negative interstitial space pressure, drawing fluid out of the capillary into the tissue (pIG = 6.3 mm Hg)

iv) The interstitial gel's colloid pressure with the same effect as pIG (pIGC = 5 mm HG).

This results, in normal situations, in the following net force at the arterial end of the capillary:

pCAP + pIGC + pIG - pCO or 25 + 5 + 6.3 - 28 = 8.3 mm Hg.

In the brain, this net driving force is only 2 mm Hg, keeping the brain rather "dry". At the venous capillary end the values are: 10 + 5 + 6.3 - 28 = -6.7 mm Hg, resulting in reabsorption pressure driving fluid from the tissue back into the blood. The mean Starling equilibrium yields a net filtration pressure of 0.3 mm Hg.

The platelet as the intermediary between the humoral composition and the endothelial cell, and the astrocyte as the intermediary between the vascular cells and the neuron, and the neuron of the autonomic nervous system as the intermediary between the central nervous system and its barriers, thus find their proper place in a chain of events, clinically known as the migraine attack.

REFERENCES

1. Ahtee, L., Boullin, D. J., and Paasonen, M. K. (1974): Brit. J. Pharmac., 52:245.
2. Amery, W. K., and Waelkens, J. (1983): Headache, 23:37.
3. Anselmi, B., Baldi, E., Casacci, F., and Salmon, S. (1980): Headache, 20:294.
4. Anthony, M. (1974): Presented at the Sixth International Migraine Symposium, London, September 1974.
5. Anthony, M., Hinterberger, H., and Lance, J. W. (1967): Arch. Neurol., 16:544.
6. Anthony, M., Hinterberger, H., and Lance, J. W. (1969): In: Research and Clinical Studies in Headache, Volume 2, edited by A. P. Friedman, pp. 29-59. Karger, Basel.
7. Bach, F. W., Blegvad, N., Fahrenkrug, J., Jensen, K., Jordal, R., and Olesen, J. (1984): Acta Neurol. Scand., (Suppl. 98), 69:28.
8. Baldi, E., Salmon, S., Anselmi, B., Spillantini, M. G. Capelli, G., Brocchi, A., and Sicuteri, F. (1982): Cephalagia, 2:77.
9. Barabas, G., Matthews, W., and Ferrari, M. (1984): Arch. Neurol., 41:871.
10. Basbaum, A. I., and Fields, H. L. (1978): Ann. Neurol., 4:451.
11. Bes, A., Comet, B., Dupui, Ph., Guell, A., Arne-Bes, M. C., and Geraud, G. (1984): In: The Pharmacological Basis of Migraine, edited by W. K. Amery, J. M. van Nueten, and W. Wauquier, pp. 202-212. Pitman Publ., London.
12. Bes, A., Geraud, G., Guell, A., and Arne-Bes, M. C. (1982): Nouv. Presse Med., 11/19:1475.
13. Blau, J. N. (1980): Brit. Med. J., 281: 658.
14. Bonham Carter, S. M., Youdim, M.-B. H., Sandler, M., Hunter, K. R., and Stern, G. M. (1974): Clin. Chim. Acta, 51:327.
15. Bonnet, G. F., and Lepreux, P. (1971): Sem. Hop. Paris, 47:2441.
16. Bottomley, J. M., Hanington, E., Jones, R. J., and Chapman, D. (1982): Headache, 22:256.
17. Bruyn, G. W. (1976): In: Clinical Neuropharmacology, Volume 1, edited by H. L. Klawans, pp. 185-213. Raven Press, New York.
18. Bruyn, G. W. (1980): Headache, 20:235.
19. Bruyn, G. W., and Ferrari, M. D. (1984): Cephalagia, 4:119.
20. Centonze, V., Brucoli, C., Macinagrossa, G., Attolini, E., Campanozzi, F., and Albano, O. (1983): Cephalagia, 3:125.
21. Coppen, A., Swade, C., Wood, K., and Carroll, J. D. (1979): Lancet, 2:914.
22. Couch, J. R., and Hassanein, R. S. (1977): Neurology, 27:843.
23. Curran, D. A., Hinterberger, H., and Lance, J. W. (1965): Brain, 88:999.

24. Curzon, G., Theaker, P., and Phillip, B. (1966): J. Neurol. Neurosurg. Psychiat., 29:85.
25. Dalessio, D. J. (1962): JAMA, 181:318.
26. D'Andrea, G., Toldo, M., Cananzi, A., and Ferro-Milone, F. (1984): Stroke, 15:271.
27. Deshmukh, S. V., and Meyer, J. S. (1977): Headache, 17:101.
28. Deshmukh, S. V., Meyer, J. S., and Mouche, R. J. (1976): Thrombos. Haemosts. (Stuttg.), 36:319.
29. Dhopesh, V. P., and Baskin, S. I. (1982): Headache, 22:165.
30. Di Giulio, A. M., Picotti, G. B., Cesura, A. M., Panerai, A. E., and Mantegazza, P. (1982): Life Sci., 30:1605.
31. Dvilansky, A., et al. (1976): Pain, 2:315.
32. Fanciullacci, M. (1979): Headache, 19:8.
33. Fanciullacci, M., Michelacci, S., Curradi, C., and Sicuteri, F. (1980): Headache, 20:99.
34. Føg-Muller, F., et al. (1978): In: Current Concepts in Migraine Research, edited by R. Greene, pp. 115-119. Raven Press, New York.
35. Gardner-Medwin, A. R. (1981): J. Exp. Biol., 95:111.
36. Gardner-Medwin, A. R. (1981): J. Physiol., 316:23P.
37. Gardner-Medwin, A. R., and Skelton, J. L. (1982): In: Cerebral Hypoxia in the Pathogenesis of Migraine, edited by F. C. Rose and W. K. Amery, pp. 127-131. Pitman, London.
38. Gawel, M., Burkitt, M., and Rose, F. C. (1974): J. Lab. Clin. Med., 83:877.
39. Gawel, M., Fettes, I., Kuzniak, S., and Edmeads, J. (1985): In: 5th International Symposium. Karger, Basel.
40. Geaney, D. P., Rutterford, M. G., Elliott, J. M., Schächter, M., Peet, K. M. S., and Grahame-Smith, D. G. (1984): J. Neurol. Neurosurg. Psychiat., 47:720.
41. Geraud, G., Guell, A., Courtade, M., Dupui, Ph., and Bes, A. (1983): Headache, 23:191.
42. Glover, V., Peatfield, R., Zammit-Pace, R., Littlewood, J., Gawel, M., Rose, F. C., and Sandler, M. (1981): J. Neurol. Neurosurg. Psychiat., 44:786.
43. Glover, V., Sandler, M., Grant, E., Rose, F. C., Orton, D., and Wilkinson, M. (1977): Lancet, 1:391.
44. Gordon, J. H., and Diamond, B. I. (1981): Biol. Psychiat., 16:365.
45. Gotoh, F., et al. (1984): Arch. Neurol., 41:951.
46. Grossman, A., and Clement-Jones, V. (1983): Clin. Endocrinol. Metabol., 12:31.
47. Hanington, E., et al. (1971): Nature (London), 230:246.
48. Hanington, E., Jones, R. J., and Amess, J. A. L. (1982): Lancet, 1:437.
49. Hanington, E., Jones, R. J., Amess, J. A. L., and Wachowicz, B. (1981): Lancet, 2:720.
50. Harik, S. I., and McGunigal, T. (1984): Ann. Neurol., 15:568.
51. Harper, A. M., MacKenzie, E. T., McCulloch, J., and Pickard, J. D. (1977): Lancet, 1:1034.

52. Hilton, B. P., and Cumings, J. N. (1972): J. Neurol. Neurosurg. Psychiat., 35: 505.
53. Hinterberger, H., et al. (1968): Clin. Sci., 34:271.
54. Hsu, L. K. G., et al. (1977): Lancet, 2:447.
55. Hsu, L. K. G., et al. (1979): T.I.N.S., pp. 116-118.
56. Jessell, Th. M. (1982): Lancet, 1:1084.
57. Johnson, E. S. (1978): Postgrad. Med. J., 54:231.
58. Jones, R. J., Forsythe, A. M., and Amess, J. A. L. (1982): In: Headache: Physiopathological and Clinical Concepts, Advances in Neurology, Volume 33, edited by M. Critchley, A. P. Friedman, S. Gorini, and F. Sicuteri, pp. 275-289. Raven Press, New York.
59. Kangasniemi, P., Riekkinen, P., and Rinne, U. K. (1972): Headache, 12:66.
60. Kimball, R. W., and Goodman, M. A. (1961): Neurology, 11:116.
61. Kohlenberg, R. J. (1982): Headache, 22:30.
62. Komatsumoto, S., Gotoh, F., Araki, N., and Gomi, S. (1983): In: Cerebrovascular Disease, edited by J. S. Meyer, et al., pp. 286-291. Excerpta Medica Congress Series 616, Amsterdam.
63. Kunkle, E. C., and Anderson, W. B. (1961): Arch. Ophthalm., 65:504.
64. Launay, J. H., Pradalier, A., and Dreux, C. (1982): Cephalagia, 2:57.
65. Launay, J. M., and Pradalier, A. (1985): Headache, 25:262.
66. Lauritzen, M., and Diemer, N. H. (1985): In: Proceedings of the Second International Headache Congress, edited by J. Olesen, P. Tfelt-Hansen, and K. Jensen, pp. 380-381. Headache, 1985, suppl. to Cephalagia, 1985.
67. Lechin, F., and van der Dys, B. (1980): Headache, 20:77.
68. Leysen, J. E., and Gommeren, W. (1984): In: The Pharmacological Basis of Migraine Therapy, edited by W. K. Amery, J. M. van Nueten, and W. Wauquier, pp. 255-266, Chapter 19. Pitman Publ., London.
69. Lindvall, O., Björklund, A., and Skagerberg, G. (1983): Ann. Neurol., 14:255.
70. Littlewood, J., Glover, V., Sandler, M., Petty, R., Peatfield, R., and Rose, F. C. (1982): Lancet, 1:983.
71. Lord, G. D. A., and Duckworth, J. W. (1978): Headache, 18:255.
72. Malmgren, R., Olsson, P., Tornling, G., and Unge, G. (1980): Thromb. Res., 18:733.
73. Marangos, P. J., Campbell, I. C., Schmechel, D. E., Murphy, D. L., and Goodwin, F. K. (1980): J. Neurochem., 34:1254.
74. Mitsui, Y., and Kochi, Y. (1962): Ophthalmologica, 144:341.
75. Monstad, P., and Lingjaerde, O. (1984): Acta Neurol. Scand., (Suppl. 98), 69:273.
76. Mosnaim, A., Chevesich, J., Wolf, M. E., and Diamond, S. (1984): Headache, 24:161.

77. Mück-Seler, D., Deanovic, Z., and Dupelj, M. (1979): Headache, 19:14.

78. Mück-Seler, D., Deanovic, Z., and Dupelj, M. (1982): In: Headache: Physiopathological and Clinical Concepts, Advances in Neurology, Volume 33, edited by M. Critchley, A. P. Friedman, S. Gorini, and F. Sicuteri, pp. 257-264. Raven Press, New York.

79. Olesen, J., and Lauritzen, M. (1984): In: The Pharmacological Basis of Migraine Therapy, edited by W. K. Amery, J. M. van Nueten, and W. Wauquier, pp. 7-18. Pitman Publ., London.

80. Oxman, Th. E., Hitzemann, R. J., and Smith, R. (1982): Headache, 22:261.

81. Peatfield, R. C., Gawel, M. J., Guthrie, D. L., Pearson, T. C., Glover, V., Littlewood, J., Sandler, M., and Rose, F. C. (1982): J. Neurol. Neurosurg. Psychiat., 45:826.

82. Pradalier, A., and Launay, J. M. (1982): Lancet, 1:862.

83. Rydzewski, W., and Wachowicz, B. (1978): In: Current Concepts in Migraine Research, edited by R. Greene, pp. 153-158. Raven Press, New York.

84. Sandler, M., Youdim, M. B., and Hanington, E. (1974): Nature, London, 250:335.

85. Sicuteri, F. (1972): Headache, 12:69.

86. Sicuteri, F. (1973): Headache, 13:19.

87. Sicuteri, F. (1977): Headache, 17:129.

88. Sicuteri, F. (1982): In: Headache: Physiopathological and Clinical Concepts, Advances in Neurology, Volume 33, edited by M. Critchley, A. P. Friedman, S. Gorini, and F. Sicuteri, pp. 65-74. Raven Press, New York.

89. Sicuteri, F. (1983): Cephalagia, 3:187.

90. Sicuteri, F., Boccuni, M., Fanciullacci, M., D'Egidio, P., and Bonciani, M. (1982): In: Headache: Physiopathological and Clinical Concepts, Advances in Neurology, Volume 33, edited by M. Critchley, A. P. Friedman, S. Gorini, and F. Sicuteri, pp. 199-208. Raven Press, New York.

91. Sicuteri, F., Boccuni, M., Fanciullacci, M., and Gatto, G. (1983): Headache, 23:179.

92. Sicuteri, F., Spillantini, M. G., Panconesi, A., and Cangi, F. (1984): In: The Pharmacological Basis of Migraine Therapy, edited by W. K. Amery, J. M. van Nueten, and W. Wauquier, pp. 171-188, Chapter 13. Pitman Publ., London.

93. Sicuteri, F., Testi, A., and Anselmi, B. (1961): Int. Arch. Allergy Appl. Immuno., 19:55.

94. Somerville, B. W. (1975): Neurology, 25:239.

95. Somerville, B. W. (1975): Neurology, 25:245.

96. Somerville, B. W. (1976): Neurology, 26:41.

97. Southren, A. L., and Christoff, N. (1962): J. Lab. Clin. Med., 59:320.

98. Spierings, E. L. H. (1980): The pathophysiology of the migraine attack. Thesis, Rotterdam.
99. Symon, L., et al. (1984): In: Cerebral Ischemia, edited by A. Bes, et al., pp. 63-71. Excerpta Medica, Amsterdam.
100. Thomas, D. V. (1982): In: Headache: Physiopathological and Clinical Concepts, Advances in Neurology, Volume 33, edited by M. Critchley, A. P. Friedman, S. Gorini, and F. Sicuteri, pp. 279-281. Raven Press, New York.
101. Vardi, J., Flechter, S., Ayalon, D., Cordova, T., and Oberman, Z. (1981): Headache, 21:14.
102. Waelkens, J. (1984): Cephalagia, 4:85.
103. Wainscott, G. (1978): In: Current Concepts in Migraine Research, edited by R. Greene, pp. 105-109. Raven Press, New York.
104. Willoughby, J. (1981): Lancet, 1:445.

The Management of Headache, edited
by F. Clifford Rose. Raven Press,
New York © 1988.

COMPLICATED MIGRAINE

J. D. Carroll, MD, FRCP, FRCPE, FRCPI

Consultant Neurologist, Regional Neurological Unit, and
Reader in Clinical Neurology, University of Surrey,

and

J. A. Gray, MA, MB, BS, MRCP (UK)

Research Registrar in Neurology, Regional Neurological Unit, and
Associate Lecturer, University of Surrey,
Guildford, Surrey, England

The term complicated migraine has been used in different ways but we share the views of Lance (13) and Bickerstaff (1) that it should be reserved for cases in which the neurological symptoms and signs persist for 24 hours or more after cessation of the migraine headache. Permanent defects of cerebral function may accrue which can be of hemispheric, brainstem, or retinal origin. Fortunately, the condition is uncommon but there are no reliable statistics as to its frequency.

Fere (4) stated that Charcot believed that any of the transient disturbances of cerebral function during a migraine attack such as hemianopia, hemiplegia and aphasia could become permanent, and noted that a hemianopia was the commonest permanent sequel of an attack. The subsequent literature confirms Fere's original observation that the occipital cortex is more often involved than the rest of the nervous system. Fere (5) later stated that the cerebral blood vessels which were temporarily constricted during attacks of migraine might become permanently spastic and eventually thrombose, leading to cerebral infarction. Galezowski (6) (1881) in a paper entitled "Ophthalmic Megrim", quoted four personal cases of permanent visual defects arising as a result of an attack of migraine and two of these cases were in their teens. He had no doubt that an attack of migraine could produce a permanent defect in the nervous system. In relatively recent times, Pearce (17) produced a classification of complicated migraine which included cluster headaches, ophthalmoplegic and familial hemiplegic migraine and migraine of the basilar artery type. We would now like to suggest a classification as follows:

TABLE 1.   Complicated Migraine
                                  Permanent Defects

1.   Cortical and Subcortical
        Hemianopia
        Hemianesthesia or hemiplegia
2.   Brain Stem
        Infarction
3.   Oculomotor Palsies (Ophthalmoplegia)
4.   Retinal
        Vascular occlusion
        Ischemic papillopathy
        Central serous retinopathy

The hemianopias can be partial or complete, as in the following example:

The patient, a 37 year old housewife, had suffered from common migrain since she was a teenager. It became classical in type when she began to take the contraceptive pill in her twenties. Despite stopping the pill, her migraine continued to be classical although much less frequent, with focal features in the left field of vision. Then early one morning she felt giddy and unsteady, and this was followed by paresthesias in her left arm and an inability to see properly in her left field of vision. This was followed by severe headache. The headache subsided, but she was unable to see to her left. Clinical examination showed that she had a left homonymous hemianopia. The CT scan showed a right occipital lobe infarct and there was no change in its appearance after six weeks.

Monocular visual loss after an attack of migraine may be caused by retinal arterial occlusion and rarely by ischemic papillopathy or central serous retinopathy. The following case history is an interesting example of retinal arterial occlusion.

The patient, a 34 year old Ward Clerk had suffered from classical migraine since the age of six. The present attack commenced with visual disturbances in her left eye, which was followed by complete blindness in the same eye. Ten minutes later she experienced right sided headache and vomiting. She did not recover the sight in her left eye. Fundal examination showed the typical features of a retinal artery occlusion.

It is our experience that hemiplegic attacks are rare, while hemisensory ones are relatively common. Repeated hemisensory attacks may leave the patient with a vague impairment of sensation down the appropriate side of the body, but detailed investigations of such cases including CT scans invariably are normal. If, however, there are neurological signs following repeated hemisensory, and especially hemiplegic attacks, then CT scan is likely to show evidence of infarction.

Permanent defects may occur in relation to basilar artery migraine but in our experience they are surprisingly uncommon, although patients with persistent diplopia might be included in this category.

Ophthalmoplegic migraine is an uncommon condition which can happen in all age groups, occurring usually in patients who had common or classical migraine for many years or as the first manifestation of the disorder. It is the term applied to recurrent attacks of unilateral headache associated with partial or complete paralysis, the latter appearing some hours after the onset of the headache or with the subsidence of the attack. The ocular palsies are transient or short lived at first, but with later attacks the paralysis may persist for days or months, and rarely may become permanent.

We have reviewed 20 cases of ophthalmoplegic migraine who have attended the Neurological Unit over the last 18 years.

TABLE 2. Ophthalmoplegic Migraine
Review of 20 Cases

3rd nerve	10 cases
3rd, 4th, and 6th nerves	
Complete external ophthalmoplegia	2 cases
3rd and 6th nerves	1 case
4th nerve	2 cases
6th nerve	1 case
Fixed pupil	4 cases

TABLE 3. Analysis of Permanent Cranial Nerve Palsies

Patient	Sex	Nerve	Number of Attacks Prior to Onset of Permanent Palsy
1	F	3rd	16
2	F	3rd	11
3	M	3rd	12
4	F	Fixed Pupil	9
5	M	Fixed Pupil	13

Those cases with a residual fixed dilated pupil had other features of a 3rd nerve palsy initially, which then recovered.

TABLE 4.   Cerebrospinal Fluid Findings
in Two Cases of Permanent Ocular Palsy Due to Migraine

Patient	Sex	Nerve	Day	Pressure	Protein mg /100ml	Cells (P.L.) /c.m.m.	
1	M	3rd	2	Normal	120	0	18
			6	Normal	35	0	2
2	F	3rd	2	Normal	95	0	20
			5	Normal	30	0	3

It should be noted that in both cases the protein content of the
fluid was raised when the lumbar puncture was performed on the
second day following the development of the paralysis, but the
content was within normal limits when the puncture was repeated
a few days later.

The ocular paresis could be caused by direct vascular
compression or by interference with the flow in the vasa
nervorum (20). Vijayan (19) supported the latter opinion and so
the condition could be regarded as a delayed ischemic
neuropathy.

In recent years there have been reports of permanent
defects following preventive therapy with propranolol in
patients with focal features in their migraine (8,18). This
could possibly be a result of hypotension or excessive
vasoconstriction during an already ischemic phase but it is not
possible, from a study of the case reports, to exclude the
neurological deficit in these cases being produced by an
alternative vascular lesion.

Oral contraceptives have been linked with permanent defects
and it is now considered inadvisable to use this form of
contraception in women whose headaches are associated with focal
neurological features, especially if over the age of thirty.

In considering the possible relationship between
complicated migraine and transient ischemic attacks there are
some who argue against the very existence of complicated
migraine, claiming that these episodes are due to embolism or
thrombosis rather than vascular spasm. Indeed, in the older
group of patients presenting with headache and focal
neurological features with no past history of migraine, the
headache is often regarded as part of a transient ischemic
attack and treated with anti-platelet drugs such as aspirin,
rather than standard migraine prophylactics. There may well be
a considerable overlap between these two conditions in that
there is substantial evidence for increased platelet
aggregability in migraine patients before and during an attack,
as well as in headache free periods (2,9).

In two small studies aspirin either alone or in combination with dipyridamole has been used in the prophylaxis of migraine (14,16). Further studies on the use of these agents in this condition are clearly needed. Perhaps migraine and transient ischemic attacks should be seen as part of a spectrum involving vessel wall spasm and platelet aggregation. Since platelets release vasospastic substances such as serotonin both of these processes probably co-exist to a varying degree in the two conditions. Complicated attacks of migraine may then occur when excessive platelet aggregation and/or arterial spasm lead to infarction of brain tissue. Vessel thrombosis, however, need not necessarily occur.

Studies on the coronary circulation may also throw light on this topic since it has been suggested that spasm in the coronary arteries may lead to myocardial infarction in the absence of primary thrombosis (3,10). The use of calcium antagonists such as nifedipine is especially beneficial in patients with coronary artery spasm, and there is evidence that the latter drug may have a role to play in the treatment of migraine (11). Interest is also growing in the possible use of the newer agent nimodipine in this context, as it may be more selective in the cerebral circulation (7,12).

How, in the light of these studies, should one manage a patient who has had an attack of complicated migraine? The following approach would seem reasonable in the light of our present knowledge. Oral contraceptives should clearly be avoided and possibly beta blockers should not be chosen as the first line in therapy. Anti-platelet drugs, especially aspirin, could be used and, if the attacks continued to be frequent, they could be combined with standard migraine prophylactics such as cyproheptadine (Periactin) and pizotifen (Sanomigran). It should be realized in this connection that pizotifen may also have anti-platelet properties (15). It is possible that in the future calcium antagonists could play a useful role in this situation, and controlled trials on the use of anti-platelet drugs and calcium antagonists in this context would be of value in establishing the optimal long term treatment for this condition.

REFERENCES

1. Bickerstaff, E. R. (1984): In: Progress in Migraine Research, Volume 2, edited by F. C. Rose, p. 83. Pitman, London.
2. Deskmukh, S. V., and Meyer, J. S. (1977): Headache, 17:101.
3. El-Maraghi, N. R. H., and Sealey, B. J. (1980): Circulation, 61:199.
4. Fere, C. (1881): Rev. Med. Paris, 1:625.
5. Fere, C. (1883): Rev. Med. Paris, 3:194.
6. Galezowski, X. (1881): Lancet, 1:176.
7. Gelmers, H. J. (1983): Headache; 23:106.
8. Gilbert, G. J. (1982): Headache, 22:81.
9. Hanington, E. (1978): Lancet, 2:501.
10. Helmstrom, R. A. (1979): Amer. Heart J., 449.
11. Kahan, A., et al. (1983): N. Engl. J. Med., 1102.
12. Kazda, S., and Towart, R. (1982): Acta Neurochirogica, 63:259.
13. Lance, J. W. (1982): Mechanism and Management of Headache, 4th Edition, p. 128. Butterworth Scientific, London.
14. Masel, B. E., et al. (1980): Headache, 20:13.
15. Mazal, S., and Rachmilewitz, E. A. (1980): J. Neurol. Neurosurg. Psychiat., 43:1137.
16. O'Neill, B. P., and Mann, J. D. (1978): Lancet, 2:1179.
17. Pearce, J. (1969): Migraine. Charles C Thomas, Springfield.
18. Prendez, J. Z. (1980): Headache, 20: 93.
19. Vijayan, N. (1980): Headache, 20:300.
20. Walsh, J. G., and O'Doherty, S. S. (1960): Neurology, 10:1079.

The Management of Headache, edited by F. Clifford Rose. Raven Press, New York © 1988.

TREATMENT OF THE ACUTE ATTACK OF MIGRAINE

Marcia Wilkinson, MA, DM, FRCP

The City of London Migraine Clinic, 22 Charterhouse Square, London EC1M 6DX, England

Treatment should be started as soon as possible in the attack because with the correct therapy the attack may be aborted in the early stages but, even if treatment is not started until the attack is well under way, it may still be effective. Some patients know the night before that they may be getting an attack and if there are any prodromal symptoms, such as a slight headache or a change in mood, treatment with metoclopramide or domperidone, and aspirin or paracetamol, should be taken then.

Rest

Rest plays an important part in the treatment of migraine (15) and sufferers should if possible lie down in a quiet dark room. Those who can go to sleep recover more quickly than do those who only rest and doze. Sometimes even 10 or 15 minutes of sleep help, but most people seem to need 2-3 hours.

Anti-Nauseants

The majority of migraine suffers (95%) also have nausea and vomiting (12), and 20% have diarrhoea. Metoclopramide (10 mg) is the drug of choice because not only is it a good anti-nauseant but it also promotes normal gastro-intestinal activity. Many migraineurs suffer from gastric stasis and the metoclopramide should be taken at the onset of the first symptom, other treatment being taken 10 to 15 minutes later. Metoclopramide is best given by injection (4), but most people find that it is also helpful taken by mouth or suppository (5). One-hundred-fifty patients attending a migraine clinic in Copenhagen (11) were treated either with metoclopramide (10 mg intramuscularly, 20 mg by suppository) or with a placebo in a double blind trial. All the patients simultaneously or 30 minutes later received paracetamol (1000 mg) and diazepam (5 mg) by mouth. The nausea was relieved in 71% by placebo and bed-rest, but metoclopramide was significantly more effective and

relieved nausea in 86%. Metoclopramide by itself did not reduce
the pain, but enhanced the effect of the analgesic or sedative
medication. Metoclopramide may cause extrapyramidal symptoms,
particularly in children, and should not usually be given to
those under ten years old. If side effects do occur, they are
usually transitory. Recently domperidone, also a potent
antagonist of dopamine receptors, has been found useful and, as
it is thought not to cross the blood brain barrier, it is less
likely to cause side effects.

Other anti-emetics such as prochlorperazine or cyclizine
can be used but they are not so effective as they tend to
depress gastrointestinal activity.

Analgesics

Aspirin (600-900 mg) or paracetamol (1000 mg) are the drugs
of choice. Aspirin, possibly because of its antiprostaglandin
effect, is probably the best but should not be used by those who
have any history of gastro-intestinal upset or bleeding
tendency. Many sufferers find that a particular proprietary
preparation suits them, and if this is so they should be
encouraged to use it. These preparations may contain either
aspirin or paracetamol combined with a small amount of codeine
and, in the U.K., combinations of paracetamol with an
antihistamine and codeine such as Migraleve, or with a
sympathomimetic and sedative such as Midrid, are popular. Where
possible, soluble or effervescent preparations such as Claridin
or Paragesic should be used, as they are more quickly absorbed.
Various studies (7,8) have been done to show the efficacy of
different preparations.

There are now on the market preparations such as Migravess
(aspirin and metoclopramide) and Paramax (paracetamol and
metoclopramide) but there is no evidence that they are better
than the drugs taken separately, and they are more expensive.

Ergotamine Tartrate

Ergotamine tartrate was first used for the treatment of
migraine in the 1920's and since then many people have shown it
to be useful. It is, however, not essential and over half of
migraine sufferers do not need it in the attack. The toxic dose
is not much greater than the therapeutic dose, and in the past
there has been a tendency to give too much. The correct dose is
probably between one and two milligrams per attack, and the
maximum that should be used in one week is 6 mg. The situation
is further complicated by the fact that the bioavailability of
ergotamine tartrate differs considerably from one individual to
another. Ala-Hurula (1) in a recent study found that in 20% of
migraineurs the treatment was unsuccessful, and that in only 36%
was the response good. In another study (2) he found that in
nine patients with a moderate, and three with a poor, response,
the mean plasma level stayed below 0.10ng/ml and that the peak

occurred at three hours. In the good responders there is usually a plasma ergotamine level of 0.20 ng/ml with a peak at one hour. This difference in absorption was also shown by Orton (9), the biggest difference being shown in volunteers who were given cafergot suppositories. Recent work at the City of London Migraine Clinic has shown that absorption by rectum or inhalation is usually better than when ergotamine tartrate is given by mouth. Earlier studies by Ala-Hurula (2) and his colleagues showed that the highest plasma levels of ergotamine tartrate were obtained after intramuscular injection, but this preparation is no longer available in the U.K.

Ergotamine Tartrate Poisoning

The early signs of ergotamine tartrate poisoning are nausea, vomiting, headache, and a feeling of not being very well (10,13), very similar symptoms to those of a migraine attack. It is because of this that many people continue to take ergotamine tartrate in their attacks, and this creates a vicious circle, particularly as the toxic symptoms appear to be alleviated by more ergotamine tartrate. In an interesting study, Ala-Hurula (3) and his colleagues gave ten subjects 2 mg ergotamine tartrate daily for three days. One to two hours after the first dose there was a peak plasma level of 0.35 ng/ml, but then the level did not rise until after the third dose when the plasma ergotamine level began to rise slowly, reaching a maximum on the sixth day. The authors considered that this supported the concept of accumulation of the drug or of immunoreactive metabolites, and concluded that in a significant number of patients who use the drug daily, ergotamine tartrate does not appear to be biologically available.

The problem of minor overdose is considerable and, at the City of London Migraine Clinic at one time (14), 4% of the patients referred were suffering from this. The major toxic effects such as gangrene are rarely seen although in the U.K. there has recently been a case where a massive overdose was prescribed and dispensed which resulted in the patient developing gangrene of the feet.

The following is a list of the ergotamine preparations available in the U.K.:

Oral:

CAFERGOT (Wander)	ergotamine tartrate 1 mgm
	caffeine 100 mgm
MIGRIL (Wellcome)	ergotamine tartrate 2 mgm
	cyclizine hydrochloride 50 mgm
	caffeine 100 mgm

Sublingual:

LINGRAINE (Winthrop)	ergotamine tartrate 2 mgm

Suppositories:
<u>Suppositories:</u>

          CAFERGOT (Wander)   ergotamine tartrate 2 mgm
                                   caffeine 100 mgm

<u>Inhalation:</u>

          MEDIHALER (Riker)   ergotamine 360 micrograms
                                   metered inhalation

In the U.K. ergotamine injections have been withdrawn, but dihydro-ergotamine mesylate (Dihydergot) is available as an injection 1-2 mgm.

Effergot, half or one tablet, was probably the best oral preparation (2), but this too is no longer available. If vomiting occurs early in the attack, a half or one Cafergot suppository should be used. Inhalation (Riker Medihaler) is an efficient way of taking ergotamine tartrate and has the advantage that the dose can be monitored easily (0.36 mg/puff) but many patients find this preparation nauseating after continued use.

To sum up, the best treatment for an acute attack is sleep, an effective anti-nauseant, preferably metoclopramide, and an analgesic, aspirin or paracetamol, and 1 or 2 mgs of ergotamine tartrate. This is the treatment that has been used at the City of London Migraine Clinic for the last seven years, during which time over 4,000 patients with acute headaches have been treated.

REFERENCES

1. Ala-Hurula, V. (1982): Europ. J. Clin. Pharmacol., 21:397.
2. Ala-Hurula, V., Myllylä, V. V., Arvela, P., Heikkilä Kärki, N., and Hokkanen, E. (1979): Europ. J. Clin. Pharmacol., 15:51.
3. Ala-Hurula, V., Myllylä, V. V., Arvela, P., Karki, N. T., and Hokkanen, E. (1979): Europ. J. Clin. Pharmacol., 16:355.
4. Bateman, D. N., and Davies, D. S. (1979): Lancet, 1:166.
5. Bateman, D. N., Kahn, C., and Davies, D. S. (1979): J. Clin. Pharmacol., 19:371.
6. Graham, A. M., Johnson, E. S., Persaud, N. P., Turner, P., and Wilkinson, M. (1984): In: Progress in Migraine Research, Volume 2, edited by F. C. Rose. Pitman, London.
7. Hakkarainen, H., Gustafsson, B., Pharm, M., and Stockman, O. (1978): Headache, 18:35.
8. Hakkarainen, H., Quiding, H., and Stockman, O. (1980): J. Clin. Pharmacol., 20:590.
9. Orton, D. A., and Richardson, R. J. (1982): Postgrad. Med. J., 58:6.
10. Rowsell, A. R., Neylan, C., and Wilkinson, M. (1973): Headache, 13:65.
11. Tfelt-Hansen, P., Olesen, J., Aebelholt-Krabbe, A., Melgaard, B., and Veilis, B. (1980): J. Neurol. Neurosurg. Psychiat., 43:369.
12. Volans, G. N.: Brit. J. Clin. Pharmacol., 2:57.
13. Wilkinson, M. (1980): J. Drug Res., 5:44.
14. Wilkinson, M., Neylan, C., and Rowsell, A. (1973): Background to Migraine, Symposia, pp. 143-149.
15. Wilkinson, M., Williams, K., and Leyton, M. (1978): Research and Clinical Studies in Headache. Headache Today - An Update by 21 Experts, pp. 141-146. S. Karger, Basel.

The Management of Headache, edited
by F. Clifford Rose. Raven Press,
New York © 1988.

PROPHYLACTIC THERAPY

F. Clifford Rose, FRCP

Director, Princess Margaret Migraine Clinic,
Department of Neurology,
Charing Cross Hospital, London W6 8RF England

and

R. Peasfield, MD, MRCP

Senior Registrar, Department of Neurology,
Leeds General Infirmary, Leeds, England

In the absence of a satisfactory animal model for migraine, one way to attempt to understand its pathogenesis is to make deductions from the pharmacological properties of drugs proven to be of clinical value. Our present understanding of these properties differs in many cases from the rationale that initially led to the use of each drug (38), and the value of many drugs (e.g., propranolol) was discovered by chance. In this chapter we shall concentrate on the evidence of each drug's clinical efficacy and on present understanding of which pharmacological properties are likely to be responsible. It is particularly important to emphasize those actions evident at clinically appropriate drug concentrations. The need for further pharmacological studies will become obvious.

The first problem is the definition of migraine, which is considered in Chapter 1. Few clinically oriented research workers emphasize the crucial importance of the diagnostic criteria used: thus every clinical trial must be critically examined in the light of the probability that patients with other types of headaches are being included. A drug whose major action is anxiolytic may prove beneficial only because the series includes patients with psychogenic headache.

Most clinicians rely on the criteria of the "Ad Hoc Committee on Classification of Headache" of the United States National Institute of Neurological Diseases and Blindness (2). This defines vascular headaches as predominantly unilateral, usually associated with anorexia and sometimes with nausea and vomiting: some are preceded by a prodrome and they are often familial. That this definition is too all-embracing is only too evident. Olesen (84) regards it as "too vague to form a satisfactory basis of research", and Diehr et al. (29) state "it is difficult to create operational definitions for headache types using such criteria". Some workers doubt the validity of distinguishing unequivocally between tension headache and migraine (9,31,122), but in spite of this, a definition excluding all but the most unequivocal cases of migraine should be a sine qua non of an acceptable drug trial. Some workers (88) have argued that such trials should be done in patients with only one type of migraine, e.g., common or classical; but this would greatly reduce the number of patients recruited in any given time and any conclusions drawn could then be applied only to patients with one type of migraine.

A working definition of migraine, first introduced by Vahlquist (120), regards migrainous headaches as "recurring headache attacks separated by pain free intervals", with two of (a) nausea, (b) scotoma or related phenomena, (c) one-sided pain, and (d) positive heredity. These criteria received validation by the epidemiological studies of Bille (13), who showed that schoolchildren with paroxysmal and non-paroxysmal headaches could be distinguished most reliably by separating the children with two or more positive criteria from the rest. Vahlquist's criteria were also used by Ekbom et al. (34) in their studies of the prevalence of migraine in military recruits. The use of a subject's family history is the least satisfactory part of the definition, as it is beset with difficulties unless the affected relative can be interviewed and diagnosed. The family history was not used by Waters in his extensive studies of the prevalence of migraine in a South Wales community (122), but he showed that twice as many of his subjects fulfilled all three of the remaining criteria than would be expected by chance, and that headaches accompanied by these symptoms tended to be more severe. This lends support to a differentiation of migraine from tension headache, whilst still allowing the possibility that both are part of the same continuum.

The importance of these diagnostic criteria does not necessarily extend to clinical practice, since many analgesics are as effective for non-migrainous headaches as for typically migrainous ones, though there have been few studies in the former using specific prophylactic drugs. The diagnostic uniformity of the series of patients studied must, however, be considered when assessing each published drug trial.

GENERAL MEASURES

With the establishment of the diagnosis of migraine, it is important to reassure the patient as early as possible that there is no evidence of any progressive or life threatening disease. Many patients will respond to this alone. Prolonged fasting may be a precipitating factor in many patients, with improvement often following a more regular schedule of meals.

The "sleeping in" or weekend headache, perhaps with this as its basis, is commonly cured by maintaining the same timetable seven days a week. A proportion of patients describe attacks caused by dietary constituents, particularly chocolate, cheese, oranges, and sometimes pork, and by alcohol, sometimes only of a specific type. Others, who consume them daily, may not have noticed an association with their headache. All these patients may be improved, often greatly, if they avoid such foods (64).

Migraine nearly always remits during pregnancy, when most drugs available for its treatment should be avoided. In contrast, the condition is often greatly worsened by most, if not all, contraceptive pills (23), and it may be up to one year before the headaches subside after the contraceptive pill has been withdrawn (96). The risks of a permanent neurological deficit are increased (57,96). It is inappropriate, therefore, to give any prophylactic medication to a patient on the contraceptive pill without stopping it first, at least for a trial period.

PROPHYLACTIC MEDICATION

This is recommended for patients having two or more attacks each month. There is a place for benzodiazepines (e.g., Tranxene at night), particularly in those patients where stress appears a precipitating factor.

Clonidine

The first prophylactic agent marketed specifically for migraine, clonidine, is probably no better than placebo in the majority of patients (14,76). Some authorities, however, consider it useful in patients whose attacks are clearly linked to dietary constituents (124). The reason for these discrepancies has not always been established. Some trials alleged to establish benefit are badly flawed; for example, one (103) recruited patients from general practice, where attacks may have been milder and provided no diagnostic criteria. The trial shows benefit only in a sub-group of patients with frequent attacks, and two patients deteriorating on clonidine are excluded from analysis (83,95). Another trial (105) gave treatment for only three weeks, whilst Sjaastad and Stensrud (106) substituted placebo on a double-blind basis in a group of patients who had already "responded" to clonidine, though they were still having a mean of 5.8 attacks in a five week period.

There is no clear correlation between benefit and the dose of clonidine used, nor the duration of treatment (47); in some trials, indeed, a worsening of headaches has been reported with prolonged clonidine treatment. Patients with less frequent headaches do better in some trials (47,103), but not in others (106). The suggestion (124), based on an open study, that clonidine is effective in diet or tyramine-precipitated headache has not been confirmed (11,14,76,99).

There is, therefore, very little reliable evidence that clonidine is superior to placebo, and speculation about the pathogenesis of migraine from its known pharmacological properties would appear unwarranted.   In animal experiments, clonidine had little pharmacological activity in doses alleged to be of clinical value (38).   In contrast to methysergide, however, is the apparent enhancement by clonidine (2 ng/ml) of the vasoconstrictor action of serotonin on isolated blood vessels in vitro (39).   Even the basic premise that low doses of clonidine given chronically inhibit vascular reactivity (129) has recently been questioned.   Thus, in a detailed, well controlled study in anesthetized monkeys, Mylecharane et al. (78) found no decrease whatsoever in cranial vascular reactivity to a number of vasoactive agents, many of which have been implicated in the pathogenesis of migraine, following chronic treatment with doses of clonidine equivalent to those used in migraine.   Their conclusion that "it...is...unlikely that a direct inhibitory action on vascular smooth muscle could be responsible for any possible therapeutic efficacy of low doses of clonidine" casts doubt over both the concept and the reality of the use of clonidine in migraine.

Indoramin
The introduction of indoramin as an anti-migraine agent rests   on   the   assumption   that   noradrenaline   induced vasoconstriction, mediated through alpha adrenoreceptors in the cranial vasculature, is the fundamental factor initiating migraine attacks (59).   Recent studies of regional cerebral blood flow in migraine patients, using tomography after Xe^{133} inhalation or injection, however, have suggested that this traditional vasospastic model is too simplistic (85-87).   In these   studies   no   change   in   cerebral   blood   flow   could   be demonstrated during the early stages of common migraine (87); although   reductions   in   flow   could   be   demonstrated   during classical migraine, they were of insufficient magnitude and timing to explain the patients symptoms, and they spread across cerebral vascular territories (86).   In the light of these new findings it is not too surprising that indoramin has yet to be shown to be an important clinical advance.

Pizotifen
The drugs of first choice are pizotifen and propranolol. Pizotifen is considered to block 5-hydroxytryptamine receptors, though it may also have a partial agonist action. In a dose of 0.5 mg t.d.s., increasing if necessary to 1 mg t.d.s., it produces a significant improvement in about 70% of patients (8,72,92), but some of these relapse after six months or more on the drug. The principal side effect is increased appetite with a tendency to gain weight, which may cause some female patients to insist on alternative treatment despite improvement. It can also induce drowsiness.

Propranolol

Propranolol is much the most effective of the beta blockers in treating migraine (28,123); timolol has some beneficial action (16), but alprenolol (33), acebutolol (80), and pinolol (106) very little. From these observations it seems likely that the improvement with propranolol is due to an action independent of beta blockade. Further support for this idea comes from the results of a trial of D-propranolol (113) which retains the membrane stabilizing properties of L-propranolol while having no action at beta receptors. This drug is almost as effective a prophylactic agent in migraine as DL-propranolol, the form in common use (112). Many patients respond to a dose of 40 mg b.d. of DL-propranolol, but some require as much as 320 mg daily (the long-acting preparation is very convenient). It is unfortunate that there is no drug of this type suitable for use in patients with a history of asthma.

Metergoline

The potent 5-HT receptor blocking activity of metergoline has been demonstrated in a number of behavioral (36,44,89), electrophysiological (102), biochemical (44,48), and peripheral (89) test systems. In common with other ergot derivatives, metergoline, at higher concentrations, displaces radioligand binding to dopamine receptors (55). Only one open trial in migraine has been reported (42), with benefit in 21 out of 37 migraine patients.

Lisuride

This drug is a semi-synthetic, ergot alkaloid with potent peripheral serotonin antagonistic properties and is also a dopaminergic agonist (55). In a double-blind multi-center trial (53), 53 patients were treated with methysergide (6 mg daily), and 72 with lisuride (75 μ g daily); 53% of the patients on lisuride, and 51% on methysergide, showed a reduction of more than 50% in the number of attacks after three months' treatment. In addition, 128 patients (58 on lisuride and 70 on methysergide) dropped out before completing the trial, largely due to side effects (nausea, vomiting, dizziness and myalgia) which were significantly more common in the methysergide treated patients.

In a further double-blind trial Somerville and Herman (108) treated 66 migraine patients with lisuride (75 μ g daily) and 66 with placebo. Before treatment 16 subjects in each group had two or fewer headaches monthly; after three months' treatment 28 patients on lisuride and 19 on placebo fell into this catogory ($p < 0.05$). Twelve patients on lisuride and 5 on placebo dropped out due to side effects (notably muscle and chest pains), while 17 on placebo and 8 on lisuride dropped out because of lack of efficacy and 7 and 8 patients respectively for other reasons.

In a similar study lasting six months (54), 37 out of 99 patients on lisuride and 28 out of 110 patients on placebo improved (reduced to two or fewer headaches per month) ($p < 0.05$), with a similar drop out rate.

Miscellaneous Drugs with 5-HT Receptor Blocking Activity

Sulman and his colleagues have provided evidence of the clinical efficacy of two agents with established 5-HT receptor blocking activity. Danitracene (9, 10-dihydro-10-1-methyl-4 piperidylidene-9-anthrol) substantially reduced the frequency of attacks in 50 out of 75 patients in a randomized, double blind trial (114). Also in a randomized, double-blind study, ORG GC94 (1, 3, 4, 14b-tetrahydro-2, 7-dimethyl-2H-dibenzo (b,g) pyrazino-(1,2-d)-(1,4)-oxazepine) almost eliminated attacks in 21 out of 30 patients (116).

Ketanserin
This is a potent displacer of radioligand binding to central $5-HT_2$ recognition sites (65,73), and blocks smooth muscle contraction induced by 5-HT in a number of tissues including blood vessels (7,32,121,125). Although it has both alpha$_1$-adrenoceptor and histamine H_1 receptor blocking properties, these occur only at concentrations some 5-40 times higher than those required to affect $5-HT_2$ receptors (7,121). Unlike methysergide, but in common with many other non-ergot 5-HT antagonists (56), ketanserin has no vasoconstrictor properties per se (121). A preliminary report suggests ketanserin may have antimigraine activity (58).

Drugs Affecting 5-HT Uptake and Metabolism

5-HT Uptake Inhibitors
Two highly selective inhibitors of 5-HT uptake into platelets and central 5-HT neurons, femoxetine and zimelidine, have recently been evaluated clinically in the prophylactic treatment of migraine. The tricyclic anti-depressant, amitriptylene is also included under this heading since, although it blocks monoamine uptake mechanisms in general, it does show some selectivity for 5-HT (68). Inhibitors of 5-HT uptake initially increase the concentration of 5-HT free in the plasma (119); subsequently, platelet 5-HT concentrations decline slowly over several weeks (15,107,117).

Femoxetine
A double-blind comparison of 20 migraine patients treated with femoxetine (300 mg daily), with 25 on placebo, showed that the benefits of the drug, in the first three months at least, were not significantly greater than that of placebo (130). In contrast, a cross-over comparison of femoxetine (400 mg daily) with propranolol (160 mg daily) in 37 patients with migraine (3) showed both drugs to reduce the number and severity of

headaches by comparison to the pre-trial period. There was no difference in the number of headaches between the two drugs, but those on propranolol treatment were less severe. Three patients experienced initial worsening of their headache on femoxetine. Eight of the patients in this trial preferred femoxetine, 16 propranolol, with 13 undecided. In a recent preliminary report, femoxetine (400 mg daily) has again been compared with propranolol (160 mg daily) in a double-blind trial (61). On this occasion, the effects of femoxetine were unremarkable; only 3 out of 24 patients claimed relief from femoxetine, whereas 11 claimed benefit from propranolol.

Zimelidine
Zimelidine, like femoxetine (3), is an antidepressant (30,52). It was superior to placebo, especially in reducing the severity of headaches in a single blind trial on 10 patients, but the headaches were exacerbated during the first one-to-two treatment weeks (117). The drug depleted platelet serotonin levels by 78%, but only reduced the mean headache index by 36%. Severe headache has been recorded as a side effect of zimelidine treatment of phobic anxiety (35), depression (109), and chronic pain (19).

Amitriptyline
Amitriptyline alone has been studied as a migraine prophylactic drug. In a double-blind study of 20 patients, Gomersall and Stuart (45) found half the patients received 50% relief. Couch et al. (21), in an open trial on 110 patients, showed that benefit was independent of the prior psychiatric state of the patient. Sixty-three of the 110 patients gained more than 80% relief and 24 patients less than 20% relief, with only 23 patients between these extremes, which they contrast to the unimodal distribution of improvement to other drugs. In a controlled trial on 100 patients, amitriptyline (100 mg daily) was significantly superior to placebo (19).

The bicyclic antidepressant viloxazine, in contrast, caused migrainous headaches in 6 out of 30 patients involved in a psychiatric trial, and 3 of these patients had migrainous visual disturbance (10). The headaches, however, resolved with continuing treatment.

It seems fair to conclude from the evidence available that the value to migraine therapy of drugs whose primary property is inhibition of 5-HT uptake remains to be proven. The rather more consistent response achieved with amitriptyline may reflect the 5-HT receptor blocking activity of this drug, which is sufficient to be manifested at doses used clinically (40). Neither femoxetine (94) nor zimelidine (43,126) has meaningful 5-HT receptor blocking activity. It may also be relevant that both amitriptyline (27) and femoxetine (104) are effective in the treatment of so-called "tension headache". Since in practice it is difficult to preclude entirely a "tension headache" component within a particular "migraine" headache, the inconsistent effects of these agents may in part reflect a variable contribution of such factors in the different studies (see also Ref. 104). In this context, it is of interest that amitriptyline has been shown to have synergistic effects with propranolol (25,67), a drug which appears to be more effective against migraine than against tension headache (67). In addition, both amitriptyline and imipramine have direct analgesic properties (110).

Monoamine Oxidase Inhibitors
Anthony and Lance (4) reported an open study of phenelzine in 25 migraine patients. In 20 of these, the headache frequency was improved by more than 50%, and the remainder reported their headaches to be less severe. The clinical response could not be correlated with the rise in plasma serotonin.

L-Tryptophan
Kangasniemi et al. (60) attempted to increase brain serotonin by L-tryptophan to 8 migraine patients, in a double-blind cross-over comparison with L-leucine. In 4 of the 8 migraine patients, headaches were markedly alleviated on treatment with L-tryptophan, but the overall clinical effect was not statistically significant.

Reserpine
A single dose of reserpine will induce headaches resembling migraine when administered subcutaneously or intramuscularly (22,62) to susceptible subjects, and this is associated with a fall in blood serotonin and a rise in urinary serotonin metabolite excretion (22). More prolonged reserpine treatment, however, decreased the frequency and intensity of migraine attacks in two open trials (37,81). Nattero et al. (81) compared the effects of reserpine and placebo in a double-blind cross-over study in 18 patients; all 18 improved on reserpine, compared with only 2 on placebo ($p < 0.001$).

Methysergide
Methysergide, though still the most potent of the specific prophylactic agents, should in most cases be treated as the drug of last choice because of the risk of retroperitoneal fibrosis if treatment is continued for more than five or six consecutive months. Doses of up to 2 mg t.d.s. have been used (96).

With the exception of methysergide, there is no reason why any of the above prophylactic agents should not be maintained indefinitely, though it may be worth tailing them off after a few months to see if the patient can manage without them.

Lithium
Lithium carbonate appears to be an effective treatment for cluster headache in doses similar to those used in psychiatry, though there have been no formal double-blind studies (90). There is, however, controversy about the effectiveness of

lithium in the treatment of migraine. Nieper (82) administered lithium orotate (750-900 mg) to 44 patients with headache in an open trial, of which 39 found the treatment to be "thoroughly effective"; he suggests that the orotic acid carrier raised intracellular lithium levels. Chazot et al. (17) administered 9.92 milli-equivalents of lithium as gluconate twice daily to 25 migraine patients (defined by ad hoc criteria) for two months, and placebo for two months, in a double-blind cross-over trial. There were significantly fewer attacks in the lithium treatment period and the patients with the greatest number of attacks showed the greatest improvement. Medina and Diamond (71) administered an average of 900 mg of lithium carbonate to 27 patients with "cyclical migraine", reporting complete remission in 5 patients and improvement in 14, and they could find no evidence of lithium being more effective in the patients with the shorter headaches (70). In contrast, Kudrow (63) reported prolonged throbbing occipital headache during lithium treatment of cluster headache, and Peatfield and Rose (91) reported that the headaches of 5 migraine patients given lithium carbonate (800-1200 mg) became more frequent and more severe, and one of their cluster headache patients developed a classical migrainous visual disturbance.

The different responses observed by these authors may relate to the different salts of lithium used, the different doses of elemental lithium (though those used by Chazot et al. (17) and by Peatfield and Rose (91) were almost identical), or to lithium being given for longer in more successful trials. Some of the patients described by Medina and Diamond (71) may have had atypical cluster headache. Further studies of lithium in migraine would appear justified.

Little of precision can be said of the mechanism of action of lithium in migraine since the ion causes numerous neurochemical changes which vary markedly with dose, mode, and duration of administration and species studied (46). In view of the generally suggested role of 5-HT in the etiology of migraine, it bears emphasis that prominent amongst these neurochemical changes are effects on the synthesis, release and uptake of 5-HT and on the sensitivity of the receptors mediating 5-HT neurotransmission (118).

Dipyramidole

The disturbance of platelet function found in migraine (for reviews see references 41 and 50) suggested that platelet inhibitory drugs might be effective in migraine prophylaxis. Dipyramidole is a phosphodiesterase inhibitor, and the resultant increase in platelet cyclic AMP potentiates prostacyclin, thus inhibiting platelet aggregation in vivo, especially when taken in conjunction with aspirin (75).

Hawkes (51) embarked on a double-blind cross-over comparison of dipyramidole (100 mg four times a day) and placebo in migraine, but all the first 9 patients reported an increase in frequency and severity of headache, coming on within the first four days of treatment in four cases. Headache has also been reported when dipyramidole is administered for transient ischemic attacks (1).

A combination of aspirin (325 mg twice daily) and dipyramidole (25 mg three times daily) was compared with placebo in a double-blind cross-over trial in 25 migraine patients (66). There was a statistically significant reduction in the frequency and intensity of headache in the treated group (p<0.05). In a four-arm trial, dipyramidole (75 mg four times daily), aspirin (325 mg four times daily), both of these, or placebo, were given to 160 migraine patients; the results suggested that the combination was the most effective and that dipyramidole alone may be associated with an initial worsening of headache, though no statistical analysis is provided (100).

Antihistamines

Although the intravenous administration of histamine will induce headache, well conducted trials of combined H1 and H2 blockade with chlorpenramine and cimetidine have shown that these agents have no prophylactic value in migraine (6,79).

Oral Contraceptives

Headache was a side-effect of oral contraception in 38% of 534 women answering an appeal for information (23). The accentuation of pre-existing migraine and de novo onset of headache are both found (12). Other patients develop focal aura symptoms for the first time: the mortality rate from cerebral thrombosis, hemorrhage and embolism is approximately doubled in women who have ever taken oral contraceptives (97), and Bickerstaff (12) found that 6 of his 62 patients suffering such events had experienced a change in pattern of their migraine immediately before the stroke. A similar excess of stroke patients with prior classical migraine was reported by Salmon et al. (101). When oral contraceptives are stopped, improvement may continue for some months (49). Relief of migraine over a longer time span than the seven day period between pill cycles has been reported, but it is so unusual that hormones cannot be recommended in the management of migraine (12). Stilbestrol has been noted to increase headaches in a 75 year old male (24).

The mode of action of contraceptive steroids in headache has not been established, although they increase platelet aggregability (49,69,93), perhaps by decreasing prostacyclin production (127).

Anticonvulsants

Carbamazepine when used for migraine has been disappointing in open studies (5). No formal studies of phenytoin have been published but there have been many anecdotal reports of its benefit, especially in children (74,96).

A non-sedative barbiturate derivative, proxibarbal, was found to be effective in a double-blind cross-over trial in 35 assorted migraine and headache patients (115); these authors speculated that the drug induces the hepatic enzymes that metabolize serotonin and histamine.

Isometheptine
Isometheptine is an indirectly acting sympathomimetic amine, which causes vasoconstriction, particularly at arteriovenous anastomoses (111).

The combination of isometheptine (65 mg) with paracetamol (325 mg) and dichloralphenazone (100 mg) (Midrin) has been shown to be more effective than placebo in mild to moderate migraine attacks (26,128). Isometheptine alone was compared with Midrin and placebo in a double-blind trial in 60 migraine patients, and both drugs were found to be superior to placebo. There were no significant differences between them, implying that isometheptine is an active constituent of the compound preparation (98).

Antihistamines, of both the H1 and H2 varieties, even given simultaneously, have been shown not to influence migraine (6). Sodium chromoglycate (Nalcrom) may be of value in diet associated migraine (20,77).

REFERENCES:

1. Acheson, J., Danta, G., and Hutchinson, E. C. (1969): Brit. Med. J., 1:614.
2. Ad Hoc Committee (1962): Classification of Headache. JAMA, 179:717.
3. Andersson, P. G., and Petersen, E. N. (1981): Acta Neurol. Scandinav., 64:280.
4. Anthony, M., and Lance, J. W. (1969): Arch. Neurol., 21:263.
5. Anthony, M., Lance, J. W., and Somerville, B. (1972): Med. J. Australia, 1:1343.
6. Anthony, M., Lord, G. D. A., and Lance, J. W. (1978): Headache, 18:261.
7. Awouters, F., Leysen, J. E., De Clerck, F., and Van Nueten, J. M. (1982): In: 5-Hydroxytryptamine in Peripheral Reactions, edited by Fred de Clerck and Paul M. Vanhoutte, pp. 193-197. Raven Press, New York.
8. Bademosi, O., and Osuntokun, B. O. (1978): Practitioner, 220:325.
9. Bakal, D. A., and Kaganov, J. A. (1979): Headache, 19:285.
10. Barnes, T. R. E., Kidger, T., and Greenwood, D. T. (1979): Lancet, 2:1368.
11. Barrie, M. A., Carpenter, M. E., Carroll, J. D., Knowlson, P. A., Neylan, C., Ross, O., Rowsell, A. R., and Wilkinson, M. I. P. (1971): In: Proceedings of the Internat. Headache Symposium, Elsinore, Denmark, edited by D. Dalessio, et al., pp. 23-26. Sandoz, Basle.
12. Bickerstaff, E. R. (1975): In: Neurological Complications of Oral Contraceptives, pp. 81-86. Clarendon Press, Oxford.
13. Bille, B. (1962): Acta Paediatr. Stockh., 51:1 Suppl. 136.
14. Boisen, E., Deth, S., Hubbe, P., Jansen, J., Klee, A., and Leunbach, G. (1978): Acta Neurol. Scandinav., 58:288.
15. Børup, C., Petersen, I.-M., Honore, P. Le F., and Wetterberg, L. (1979): Psychopharmacology, 63:241.
16. Briggs, R. S., and Millac, P. A. (1979): Headache, 19:379.
17. Chazot, G., Chauplannaz, G., Biron, A., and Schott, B. (1979): La Nouvelle Presse Medicale, 8:2836.
18. Clarke, I. M. C. (1982): Brit. Med. J., 285:1425.
19. Couch, J. R., and Hassanein, R. (1979): Arch. Neurol., 36:695.
20. Couch, J. R., and Ziegler, D. K. (1978): Headache, 18:219.
21. Couch, J. R., Ziegler, D. K., and Hassanein, R. (1976): Neurology, 26:121.
22. Curzon, G., Barrie, M., and Wilkinson, M. I. P. (1969): J. Neurol. Neurosurg. Psychiat., 32:555.
23. Dalton, K. (1976): Headache, 15:247.
24. Damasio, H., and Corbett, J. J. (1981): Ann. Neurol., 9:92.

25. Dexter, J. D., Byer, J. A., and Slaughter, J. R. (1980): Headache, 20:157.
26. Diamond, S. (1976): Headache, 15:282.
27. Diamond, S., and Baltes, B. J. (1971): Headache, 11:110.
28. Diamond, S., and Medina, J. L. (1976): Headache, 16:24.
29. Diehr, P., Diehr, G., Koepsell, R., Wood, R., Beach, K., Wolcott, B., and Tompkins, R. K. (1982): J. Chron. Dis., 35:623.
30. Drug and Therapeutics Bulletin (1982): 20:95-96.
31. Drummond, P. D. (1982): Cephalagia, 2:157.
32. Eccles, N. K., Grimmer, A. J., and Leathard, H. L. (1981): Brit. J. Pharmacol., 74:831
33. Ekbom, K. (1975): Headache, 15:129.
34. Ekbom, K., Ahlborg, B., and Shele, R. (1978): Headache, 18:9.
35. Evans, L., Best, J., Moore, G., and Cox, J. (1980): Prog. Neuropsychopharmacol., 4:75.
36. Ferrini, R., and Glasser, A. (1965): Psychopharmacologia, Berlin, 8:271.
37. Fog-Møller, F., Bryndum, B., Dalsgaard-Nielsen, T., Genefke, I. K., and Nattero, G. (1976): Headache, 15:275.
38. Fozard, J. R. (1975): J. Pharm. Pharmacol., 27:297.
39. Fozard, J. R. (1976): Europ. J. Pharmacol., 36:127.
40. Fozard, J. R. (1982): In: Headache: Physiopathological and Clinical Concepts, Advances in Neurology, Volume 33, edited by M. Critchley, A. P. Friedman, S. Gorini, and F. Sicuteri, pp. 295-307. Raven Press, New York.
41. Fozard, J. R. (1982): Prog. Pharmacol., 4:135.
42. Franchi, G., and Fanciullacci, M. (1969): Minerva Medica, 60:4313.
43. Fuxe, K., Ogren, S.-O., and Agnati, L. F. (1979): Neurosci. Lett., 13:307.
44. Fuxe, K., Ogren, S.-O., Agnati, L. F., and Jonsson, G. (1978): Neurosci. Lett., 9:195.
45. Gomersall, J. D., and Stuart, A. (1973): J. Neurol. Neurosurg. Psychiat., 36:684.
46. Gottesfeld, Z. (1976): Psychopharmacologia, Berlin, 45:239.
47. Hakkarainen, H., Hokkanen, E., and Kallanranta, T. (1980): Uppsala J. Med. Sci., (Suppl. 31), 16.
48. Hamon, M., Mallat, M., Herbet, A., Nelson, D. L., Audinot, M., Pichat, L., and Glowinski, J. (1981): J. Neurochem., 36:613.
49. Hanington, E., Jones, R. J., and Amess, J. A. L. (1982): Lancet, 1:967.
50. Hanington, E., Jones, R. J., Amess, J. A. L., and Wachowicz, B. (1981): Lancet, 2:720.
51. Hawkes, C. H. (1978): Lancet, 2:153.
52. Heel, R. C., Morley, P. A., Brogden, R. N., Carmine, A. A., Speight, T. M., and Avery, G. S. (1982): Drugs, 24:169.

53. Herrmann, W. M., Horowski, R., Dannehl, K., Kramer, U., and Lurati, K. (1977): Headache, 17:54.
54. Herrmann, W. M., Kristof, M., and Hernandez, M. S. Y. (1978): J. Internat. Med. Res., 6:476.
55. Hruska, R. E., and Silbergeld, E. K. (1981): J. Neurosci. Res., 6:1.
56. Humphrey, P. P. A., Feniuk, W., and Watts, A. D. (1982): J. Pharm. Pharmacol., 34:541.
57. Irey, N., McAllister, H. A., and Henry, J. M. (1978): Neurology, 28:12.
58. Janssen Pharmaceutica (1982): Investigational New Drug Brochure, 6th edition, p. 94.
59. Johnson, E. S. (1978): Postgrad. Med. J., 54:231.
60. Kangasniemi, P., Falck, B., Langvik, V.-A., and Hyyppa, M. T. (1978): Headache, 18:161.
61. Kangasniemi, P., Nyrke, T., Lang, H., and Petersen, E. (1982): Acta Neurol. Scandinav., 65: (Suppl. 90), p. 74.
62. Kimball, R. W., and Friedman, A. P. (1961): Neurology, 11:116.
63. Kudrow, L. (1977): Headache, 17:15.
64. Lance, J. W. (1978): Mechanism and Management of Headache, Butterworths, London.
65. Leysen, J. E., Niemegeers, C. J. E., Van Nueten, J. M., and Laduron, P. M. (1981): Molec. Pharmacol., 21:301.
66. Masel, B. E., Chesson, A. L., Peters, B. H., Levin, H. S., and Alperin, J. B. (1980): Headache, 20:13.
67. Mathew, N. T. (1981): Headache, 21:105.
68. Maxwell, R. A., and White, H. L. (1978): In: Handbook of Psychopharmacology, Volume 14, Affective Disorders: Drug Actions in Animals and Man, edited by L. L. Iverson, S. D. Iversen, and S. H. Snyder, pp. 83–155. Plenum Press, New York.
69. Mazal, S. (1978): Australia & New Zealand J. Med., 8:646.
70. Medina, J. L. (1982): Arch. Neurol., 39:386.
71. Medina, J. L., and Diamond, S. (1981): Arch. Neurol., 38:343.
72. Mikropoulos, H. E. (1978): Res. Clin. Stud. Headache, 6:167.
73. Millar, J. A., Facoory, B. D., and Laverty, R. (1982): Lancet, 2:1154.
74. Millichap, J. G. (1978): Child's Brain, 4:95.
75. Moncada, S., and Korbut, R. (1978): Lancet, 1:1286.
76. Mondrup, K., and Møller, C. E. (1977): Acta Neurol. Scandinav., 56:405.
77. Monro, J., Brostoff, J., Carini, C., and Zilkha, K. (1980): Lancet, 2:1.
78. Mylecharane, E. J., Duckworth, J. W., Lord, G. D. A., and Lance, J. W. (1980): Europ. J. Pharmacol., 68:163.
79. Nanda, R. N., Arthur, G. P., Johnson, R. H., and Lambie, D. G. (1980): Acta Neurol. Scandinav., 62:90.

80. Nanda, R. N., Johnson, R. H., Gray, J., Keogh, H. J., and Melville, I. D. (1978): Headache, 18:20.
81. Nattero, G., Lisino, F., Brandi, G., Gastaldi, L., and Genefke, I. K. (1976): Headache, 15:279.
82. Nieper, H.-A. (1973): Agressologie, 14:407.
83. Nurick, S. (1972): Lancet, 1:901.
84. Olesen, J. (1978): Headache, 18:268.
85. Olesen, J. (1982): Pathologie Biologie, 30:318.
86. Olesen, J., Larsen, B., and Lauritzen, M. (1981): Ann. Neurol., 9:344.
87. Olesen, J., Tfelt-Hansen, P., Henriksen, L., and Larsen, B. (1981): Lancet, 2:438.
88. Olesen, J., Tfelt-Hansen, P., Henriksen, L., Lauritzen, M., and Larsen, B. (1982): In: Advances in Migraine Research and Therapy, edited by F. C. Rose, pp. 105-115. Raven Press, New York.
89. Ortmann, R., Bischoff, S., Radeke, E., Buech, O., and Delini-Stula, A. (1982): Arch. Pharmacol., 321:265.
90. Peatfield, R. C. (1981): J. Royal Soc. Med., 74:432.
91. Peatfield, R. C., and Rose, F. C. (1981): Headache, 21:140.
92. Peet, K. M. S. (1977): Current Med. Res. & Opinion, 5:192.
93. Peters, J. R., Elliott, J. M., and Grahame-Smith, D. G. (1979): Lancet, 2:933.
94. Petersen, E. N., Edvinsson, L., and Hardebo, J. E. (1979): Acta Pharmacol. Toxicol, 45:296.
95. Pollard, P. A., Shafar, J., Knowlson, P. A., and Tallett, E. R. (1972): Lancet, 1:1242.
96. Raskin, N. H., and Appenzeller, O. (1980): In: Major Problems in Internal Medicine, Volume 19. W. H. Saunders, Philadelphia.
97. Royal College of General Practitioners Oral Contraception Study (1981): Lancet, 1:541.
98. Ryan, R. E. (1974): Headache, 14:33.
99. Ryan, R. E., and Ryan, R. E. Jr. (1975): Headache, 14:190.
100. Ryan, R. E., and Ryan, R. E. Jr. (1982): In: Headache: Physiopathological and Clinical Concepts, Advances in Neurology, Volume 33, edited by M. Critchley, A. P. Friedman, S. Gorini, and F. Sicuteri, pp. 247-252. Raven Press, New York.
101. Salmon, M. L., Winkelman, J. Z., and Gay, A. J. (1968): JAMA, 206:85.
102. Sastry, B. S. R., and Phillis, J. W. (1977): Canadian J. Physiol. Pharmacol., 55:130.
103. Shafar, J., Tallett, E. R., and Knowlson, P. A. (1972): Lancet, 1:403.
104. Sjaastad, O. (1983): Cephalagia, 3:53.
105. Sjaastad, O., and Stensrud, P. (1971): Acta Neurol. Scandinav., 47:120.
106. Sjaastad, O., and Stensrud, P. (1972): Acta Neurol. Scandinav., 48:124.

107. Slettnes, O., Berstad, J. R., Honore, P. Le F., and Sjaastad, O. (1978): In: Proceedings of the Scandinavian Migraine Society Annual Meeting, p. 47.
108. Somerville, B. W., and Herrmann, W. M. (1978): Headache, 18:75.
109. Sommerville, J. M., McClaren, E. H., Campbell, L. M., and Watson, J. M. (1982): Brit. Med. J., 285:1009.
110. Spiegel, K., Kalb, R., and Pasternak, G. W. (1983): Ann. Neurol., 13:462.
111. Spierings, E. L. H., and Saxena, P. R. (1980): Headache, 20:103.
112. Stensrud, P., and Sjaastad, O. (1972):
113. Stensrud, P., and Sjaastad, O. (1976): Acta Neurol. Scandinav., 53:229.
114. Sulman, F. G., Pfeifer, Y., and Superstine, E. (1977): Headache, 17:203.
115. Sulman, F. G., Pfeifer, Y., and Superstine, E. (1980): Headache, 20:269.
116. Sulman, F. G., Pfeifer, Y., and Superstine, E. (1981): Arzneimittelforschung, 31:109.
117. Syvalahti, E., Kangasniemi, P., and Ross, S. B. (1979): Current Therapeutic Res., 25:299.
118. Treiser, S. L., Cascio, C. S., O'Donohue, T. L., Thoa, N. B., Jacobwitz, D. M., and Kellar, K. J. (1981): Science, 213:1529.
119. Uzan, A., Le Fur, G., Kabouche, M., and Mitrani, N. (1978): Life Sci., 23:1317.
120. Vahlquist, B. (1955): Internat. Arch. Allergy, 7:348.
121. Van Nueten, P. M., Janssen, P. A. J., Van Beek, J., Xhonneux, R., Verbeuren, T. J., and Vanhoutte, P. M. (1981): J. Pharmacol. Exper. Therapeutics, 218:217.
122. Waters, W. E. (1973): Internat. J. Epidemiol., 2:189.
123. Widerøe, T.-E., and Vigander, T. (1974): Brit. Med. J., 2:699.
124. Wilkinson, M., Neylan, C., and Rowsell, A. R. (1971): In: Proceedings of the Internat. Headache Symposium, Elsinore, Denmark, edited by D. Dalessio, et al., pp. 219–222. Sandoz, Basle.
125. Williams, R. H., and Bradley, P. B. (1983): Lancet, 1:703.
126. Wong, D. T., Bymaster, F. P., Reid, L. R., and Threlkeld, P. G. (1983): Biochem. Pharmacol., 32:1287.
127. Ylikorkala, O., Puolakka, J., and Viinikka, L. (1981): Lancet, 1:42.
128. Yuill, G. M., Swinburn, W. R., and Liversedge, L. A. (1972): Brit. J. Clin. Pract., 26: 76.
129. Zaimis, E., and Hanington, E. (1969): Lancet, 2:298.
130. Zeeberg, I., Orholm, M., Nielsen, J. D., Honore, P. Le F., and Larsen, J. J. V. (1981): Acta Neurol. Scandinav., 64:452.

The Management of Headache, edited by F. Clifford Rose. Raven Press, New York © 1988.

A CRITIQUE OF MIGRAINE THERAPY

John Fozard, PhD

Centre de Recherche, Merrell-Dow Research Institute, Strasbourg Research Center, 16 rue d'Ankara, 67084 Strasbourg-Cedex, France

It would be unrealistic to expect a marksman to hit his target if the target were hidden from view. It would be even more unrealistic to expect him to hit more than one such target with a single bullet. Yet, in essence, this is precisely the problem migraine presents to those seeking to develop drugs for the condition. Even today the pathophysiology of migraine is largely unknown; what is certain is that it is both complex and multifactorial. Under these circumstances it is perhaps not surprising that therapeutic advances have been slow, sometimes serendipitous, and in all instances have fallen short of providing truly effective remedies (Table 1).

TABLE 1. The Advent of the Principal Migraine Therapies:

ACUTE TREATMENT:

Drug:	Date:	Rationale:
Aspirin	1899	analgesic
Paracetamol	1949	analgesic
Ergotamine	1928	sympatholytic
Metoclopramide	1974	anti-emetic gastrokinetic

PROPHYLAXIS:

Methysergide	1959	5-HT antagonist
Pizotifen	1967	5-HT/histamine antagonist
Propranolol	1966	serendipity
Calcium antagonists	1981	anti-hypoxia/spasmolytic

On this basis it would be neither fair nor constructive to criticize existing therapies for being less than ideal, but the problems can be identified by seeking the key properties of the often non-selective drugs used. Such approach should provide important clues to pathophysiology and the basis for rational development of antimigraine therapies in the future. Certain assumptions as to etiology have been necessary because, despite a plethora of theories, few migrainologists would disagree that vascular elements of both the intracranial and extracranial circulation are involved, that endogenous pain producing substances are important, and that the sensation of pain is transmitted via nociceptive afferent nerve fibers to the central nervous system.

STRATEGIES OF MIGRAINE TREATMENT

Treatment strategies fall into two modes: once the attack is underway one can attempt to abort it or, more accurately, treat the symptoms; alternatively, one can treat prophylactically in an attempt to prevent the attack developing and/or to minimize breakthrough attack severity such that symptomatic treatment is more effective. Theoretically, a truly effective and non-toxic acute treatment would obviate the necessity for prophylaxis in all except perhaps the small minority of patients whose attacks are frequent (more than one per week) and disabling. It is a measure of the gap between existing acute therapies and the ideal that the prophylactic approach, often supplemented by symptomatic treatment, is a recommended strategy in situations where attacks occur more frequently than twice a month (63,87,130).

Treatments for the Acute Acttack

The important symptoms requiring treatment are headache, nausea and vomiting in common migraine and the additional symptoms of focal cerebral dysfunction in classical migraine. With the possible exception of the calcium antagonists (vide infra), there have been no routine therapies directed at the prodromal symptoms. In the absence of clearly defined etiology, it is hardly surprising that the mainstay of symptomatic treatment has been and remains analgesic agents (aspirin, paracetamol, other non-steroidal anti-inflammatory drugs) with or without anti-emetic drugs (phenothiazines, antihistamines, metoclopramide). In addition, successful treatment of the acute attack can be achieved in many patients with ergotamine which can with justification be considered selectively antimigraine (88,130).

Analgesic drugs:

The value of non-steroidal, anti-inflammatory drugs in general and aspirin and paracetamol in particular as analgesic/anti-inflammatory agents is beyond question (103). Their efficacy in migraine is borne out by the results from several controlled studies (49,89,112) and by their use as routine therapy in specialist migraine clinics (111,130), but the therapeutic response is rarely complete (89,112), and significant residual discomfort afflicts many patients. Aspirin is as effective as paracetamol (111) and tolfenamic acid (50) and, short of intolerance, there would appear to be no sound reason for preferring more expensive options.

The efficacy of non-steroidal, anti-inflammatory drugs as symptomatic treatment lends significant support to the concept of a "sterile" inflammatory response in the cranial vasculature being a key factor in the etiology of migraine (27,78). Thus, the involvement of prostanoids in the inflammatory process is established (64), as indeed is the fact that aspirin and similar drugs are analgesic and anti-inflammatory due to inhibition of the cyclo-oxygenase step in arachidonic acid metabolism (35,103).

Realistically, one might not expect more than a partial relief of symptoms with selective cyclo-oxygenase inhibitors. Prostanoids are but one class of naturally occurring inflammatory mediators, which also include histamine, 5-hydroxytryptamine, the products of lipoxygenase and various peptides, including the kinins and substance P. If the hypothesis of a "sterile" inflammatory response has merit, the combination of aspirin or similar agents with drugs affecting one or more other inflammatory mediators would be entirely logical.

Anti-emetic drugs:

In a condition in which up to 90% of patients have nausea and some 50%-75% may vomit (66,81), the use of anti-emetic drugs as adjunct therapy is entirely logical. Although drugs of the phenothiazine, antihistamine groups have been used for many years (32), the case for metoclopramide as the drug of choice for this purpose is impressive. As a dopamine D_2 receptor antagonist (99), metoclopramide has proven activity against the nausea and emesis of migraine (104,113). In addition, metoclopramide, by a mechanism not yet understood (96), increases gastrointestinal motility and speeds up gastric emptying (51,99), an action particularly relevant to migraine where gastric stasis (62) leading to reduced rates of drug absorption (117,118,121) is a common finding. In a number of studies, parenteral and oral metoclopramide has been shown to reverse the aspirin absorption deficit of acute migraine (95,122) leading to swifter resolution of headache (113,123). Essentially similar data have been reported with metoclopramide combined with tolfenamic acid (118). By contrast, triethylperazine, a representative phenothiazine anti-emetic agent, delayed both the absorption of aspirin and the clinical recovery (126).

From the foregoing, the logical conclusion is that the combination of anti-emetic and gastrokinetic activity renders metoclopramide uniquely suited to the role of adjunct to the oral analgesic therapy of migraine, but a cautionary note is appropriate: in the vast majority of cases where metoclopramide increases analgesic absorption and/or therapeutic efficacy, the drug has been given prior to, and in many cases up to 30 minutes before, the analgesic. In view of the availability of a number of combination preparations (metoclopramide plus aspirin - Migravess; metoclopramide plus paracetamol - Paramax) it may legitimately be asked whether, when given orally and concomitantly with the analgesic, the beneficial effects of metoclopramide can be demonstrated. Only one study to date has addressed this question; Tfelt-Hansen and Olesen (112) compared in a double-blind, placebo-controlled trial the effects of effervescent aspirin (650 mg) alone and co-formulated with metoclopramide (10 mg) - Migravess. They found no significant difference between aspirin and Migravess with regard to analgesic effectiveness or to antinauseant effect. The value of metoclopramide administered concomitantly with an analgesic remains for the moment at least unproven.

Ergotamine:
Although ergotamine has stood the test of time as an effective treatment for the acute attack, the drug has a number of drawbacks in practice; for instance, it has to be given at the first signs of the onset of an attack, since once the headache has developed, the drug is unlikely to be of significant benefit (19,65). A more serious disadvantage is that the drug is poorly and erratically absorbed following therapeutically practical routes of administration, namely oral, rectal, sublingual (2,85,114). Even after intramuscular administration, the biological availability is both variable and incomplete, namely less than 50% (53). In the study of Ala-Hurula (1), the time to obtain the maximum plasma ergotamine concentration (less than 1 h) and its mangitude (more than 0.2 ng/ml) were deemed critical factors in the therapeutic outcome of treatment with ergotamine. The unpredictable absorption renders consistent achievement of these criteria in individual patients difficult and may account for the surprisingly wide variations in the clinical response to ergotamine (1,26,50,127). Co-administration with caffeine improves the intestinal absorption of ergotamine (15) and is the basis for including caffeine in a number of commercial ergotamine preparations (1,65), but it has been argued (131) that the stimulant properties of caffeine are undesirable in the majority of patients who simply wish to lie down and sleep following treatment. On this basis, a more appropriate regime might be ergotamine combined with metaclopramide which results in a significantly better clinical response than that obtained with either drug given alone (48).

A further reservation about the clinical use of ergotamine concerns its potential for toxicity, particularly that related to vasoconstriction, assumed to be the basis of its therapeutic efficacy (37,65). In animal experiments, ergotamine has been shown to constrict selectively elements of the cranial vasculature (80,98,107) but, in man, widespread vasoconstriction in both the upper and lower body accompanies the administration of therapeutic doses of ergotamine to migraine patients (110). These peripheral vasoconstrictor responses to ergotamine are remarkably sustained, being prominent even 22h following 0.5 mg of the drug i.v. and 24h after 2-4 mg given rectally. The exceptionally long duration of action does not correlate with the elimination half-life for ergotamine of 1.9h (53). Since the vasospastic response to ergotamine in vitro is also maintained for many hours and cannot be reversed by washing (77,79,86), sustained vasoconstriction in vivo may have more to do with the association and slow dissociation of ergotamine from its receptor sites than with its metabolic fate and/or elimination from the plasma.

Since sustained peripheral vasoconstriction is most unlikely to be the basis of the antimigraine action of the ergotamine, it is an unnecessary and potentially dangerous property, and is the reason why ergotamine is contraindicated in patients with chronic heart disease (14), perhpheral vascular disease and hypertension (65). It is the cause of peripheral ischemia reported as a side effect of the drug (87) which, in extreme cases, can lead to gangrene. Finally, it is undoubtedly relevant to the severe peripheral ischemia occasionally seen with ergotamine in combination with methysergide (58) or propranolol (12,119). To have the beneficial effect of ergotamine without the widespread peripheral vasoconstriction presents a genuine challenge to those concerned in improving existing therapies and would represent a most important therapeutic advance.

Prophylactic Therapies

Of the wide variety of agents which have been tried as prophylactic therapy, only two classes of compound are considered to combine efficacy with side-effect potential to an extent that have established them in clinical practice; these are the 5-HT$_2$ receptor antagonists (methysergide, pizotifen) and the beta-adrenoceptor blocking agents and particularly, of course, propranolol. However, the recent spate of publications on calcium antagonists and their use in migraine emphasizes the exciting potential of these agents for prophylactic treatment, so that they are also considered in detail.

5-HT$_2$ receptor antagonists:
The two most often prescribed drugs in this class are methysergide and pizotifen, although both cyproheptadine and amitriptyline are effective in migraine (65,97), have high affinity for 5-HT$_2$ receptors (Table 2), and therefore justify inclusion under this heading. The efficacy of methysergide and pizotifen has been proven in a number of controlled trials (Table 3); as with all other approaches to therapy, the response rate falls well short of the ideal, rarely exceeding significant benefit in more than 70% of patients treated (67, Table 3).

The evidence that these agents act through blockade of $5-HT_2$ receptors rests essentially on the fact that 5-HT has long been implicated in the pathophysiology of migraine (9,37,38,102) and that all the drugs are effective at low therapeutic doses in blocking the D (45) or $5-HT_2$ (92) receptors for 5-HT (37,39). Moreover, their other properties (blockade of histamine H_1 receptors, muscarine receptors, dopaminoceptors and/or alpha-adrenoceptors) are not generally recognized as helpful in prophylaxis. Precisely which of the differently located $5-HT_2$ receptors are involved is not established, but a plausible case can be made for those close to the terminals of the 5-HT-containing raphe neurons within the cranial vasculature, activation of which can evoke the physiological and biochemical changes leading to the "sterile" inflammatory response of migraine (42,88).

TABLE 2.   Receptor Blocking Potency
of Migraine Prophylactic Agents:

	Methy-sergide	Cypro-heptadine	Pizotifen	Amitrip-tyline
$5-HT_1$	99	700	1500	1700
$5-HT_2$	12	6.5	6.5	13
Alpha$_1$	2300	100	120	22
Alpha$_2$	2600	760	480	630
H_1	1000	2.7	1.9	3.2
Dopamine	200	31	99	290
Muscarine	1000	19	23	11

Values are K_1 (nM) from radioligand binding studies using membranes prepared from various regions of rat or guinea-pig brain.

Data Source = References 33, 69, and 93.

If 5-HT$_2$ receptor blockade is in fact the key property, then pizotifen, cyproheptadine and amitriptyline may have the edge over methysergide which, even at therapeutic doses, may display vasoconstrictor properties (11,37). On the other hand, blockade of <u>central</u> 5-HT$_2$ receptors carries with it certain neuropharmacological consequences; for instance there is an increase in food intake in experimental animals (18,23), which may be the laboratory counterpart of the increased appetite and weight gain that is a troublesome side effect of the clinical use of these agents (87). Recently, a number of novel 5-HT$_2$ receptor antagonists, with considerably increased selectivity compared to existing compounds, has been developed (24,56,57). Clinical success with such compounds would bolster the idea that 5-HT$_2$ receptor blockade protects against migraine and a therapeutic response may well be obtained with fewer side effects, but the consequences of central 5-HT$_2$ receptor blockade would persist and could represent the principal drawback to this approach.

TABLE 3. <u>Comparative Effects of Migraine Prophylactic Drugs:</u>

	Data Source*	Improvement $\geqslant$50%	Patients	Studies
1. 5-HT$_2$ Receptor Antagonists:				
Methysergide	a	58%	1472	8
Pizotifen	a	51%	528	7
2. Beta-Adrenoceptor Antagonists:				
Propranolol	a+b	51%	293	9
Timolol	c	47%	197	3
Atenolol	d	51%	20	1
Metoprolol	e	38%	123	4
3. Calcium Antagonists:				
Nimodipine	a	69%	28	1
Verapamil	f	67%	12	1
Flunarizine	g	68%	202	7

*Data Source = reference numbers:
a = Reference 46.
b = References 13, 60, and 115.
c = References 20, 108, and 115.
d = Reference 36.
e = References 7, 60, 72, and 120.
f = Reference 105.
g = Reference 5.

Propranolol and other Beta-adrenoceptor antagonists:

Following anecdotal reports that patients being treated
with propranolol for angina pectoris obtained significant relief
of their migraine (94,135), there have been many sound
controlled trials in which the efficacy of propranolol as a
prophylactic agent has been established (see 88,128).   Until
relatively recently it was thought that the beneficial effects
in migraine were a feature of propranolol in particular rather
than beta-adrenoceptor antagonists in general, since a number of
other such compounds including pindolol, oxprenolol, alprenolol
and acebutalol had been shown to be of no, or at best limited,
value (88,128).   However,   it   is   now   clear   that   the
beta$_1$-adrenoceptor selective antagonists, atenolol (36,109) and
metoprolol (7,60) are also effective, as is the non-selective
antagonist timolol (20,115).   Response rates are generally
similar to those of the 5-HT$_2$ receptor antagonist drugs (Table
3) and, like them, a significant number of patients (10%-30%)
derive little benefit from treatment.   Side effects, although
numerous, are seldom severe (88).

The   success   of   some,   but   not   all,   beta-adrenoceptor
antagonists in prophylaxis raises the crucial question as to
whether beta-adrenoceptor blockade is in fact relevant to the
antimigraine effect.   Searching analyses of the properties of
the   active   and   inactive   compounds   (39,88,101,128)   have   not
provided a convincing answer, but it is clear that none of the
classical   properties   of   the   beta-adrenoceptor   antagonists
(beta-adrenoceptor blockade, selectivity of action, intrinsic
sympathomimetic activity, membrane stabilizing activity, brain
penetration) can per se explain their action in migraine.   The
striking   absence   of   clinical   efficacy   in   those   drugs   with
intrinsic sympathomimetic activity suggests that this property
may   act   adversely   to   counteract   any   beneficial   effect   in
migraine (101).

Although it is probably unwise to dismiss beta-adrenoceptor
blockade as being in some way important to the anti-migraine
effect, other explanations are certainly possible; for instance,
a   number   of   beta-adrenoceptor   antagonists   are   effective
antagonists at certain 5-HT receptors (39,101), including the
peripheral   neuronal   5-HT   receptors   implicated   in   the   pain
generation   of   the   acute   attack   (40,42).   Several
beta-adrenoceptor blocking agents have the capacity to inhibit
human platelet aggregation and thromboxane A$_2$ generation in both
in vitro (129) and, albeit in high doses, in vivo (22).

The   question   of   the   precise   mode   of   action   of   beta-
adrenoceptor blocking agents in migraine is not merely academic.
Beta-adrenoceptor blockade is the reason why propranolol is
contraindicated in asthma, heart block and heart failure (88)
and   certain   adverse   effects   such   as   exercise   intolerance,
hypotension and bradycardia (75) undoubtedly arise from this
source.   If beta-adrenoceptor blockade is not essential, then
theoretically   the   anti-migraine   effects   could   be   obtained
without these particular therapeutic problems.   An important

task for the scientific community is surely to establish beyond doubt the mode of action of the beta-adrenoceptor antagonists in migraine as the first step to the development of newer more selective therapies.

As a postscript to the use of beta-adrenoceptor antagonists in migraine, there are two reports in which propranolol has been claimed to be effective as symptomatic treatment. Tokola and Hokkanen (116) found an "excellent or good response to the medication (propranolol 40-120 mg) in 53% of the patients". Featherstone (34) claimed that in six of his cases "propranolol therapy (10-40 mg) was apparently effective in aborting acute migraine headaches, mostly in patients who had common migraine". One presumes that propranolol and the beta-adrenoceptor antagonists are used as prophylactic therapy because of the beneficial effects having been discovered during continuous administration for other cardiovascular disorders, but the data of Tokola and Hokkanen (116) and Featherstone (34), admittedly obtained under open conditions, indicate that a significant number of patients could be helped by symptomatic treatment with propranolol and possibly other beta-adrenoceptor antagonists. Intermittent treatment with such powerful drugs would be preferable to continuous long-term administration as a general principle. A more practical point would be that therapy with these agents could, in the event of symptomatic efficacy, be extended to the many patients in whom prophylactic therapy would not normally be justified. There is surely a strong case here for controlled clinical studies to seek to establish the value of selected beta-adrenoceptor antagonists in symptomatic treatment.

Calcium antagonists:
The classic theory of the vascular basis of migraine holds that a period of cerebral vasospasm severe enough to cause cerebral hypoxia and ischemia is the basis of the prodromal symptoms and that vasodilation, particularly in the extracranial vasculature, is the cause of the headache (133). The vasospastic theory of migraine is, in the light of recent studies (68,83,84) almost certainly too simplistic, but its ramifications were a key element in the introduction of so-called "calcium antagonists" into prophylaxis (3,6,90,136). Such compounds, it was reasoned, would block calcium entry into cells exposed to hypoxic conditions (3). Moreover, since an increase in extracellular "free" calcium is the final common pathway in the vasoconstriction process, calcium antagonists would be spasmolytic, irrespective of the initiating vasoconstrictor stimulus (90). The clinical trials reported to date amply confirm the enormous clinical potential of this group of compounds, but precisely how these drugs bring about their beneficial effects remains an open question.

In discussing the clinical responses to the different calcium antagonists, it is important to recognize that these compounds, although often considered together, are in fact a highly heterogeneous group. Spedding (106) has identified three classes of calcium antagonists based on physico-chemical and functional grounds (Table 4). Class 1 comprises the dihydropyridines including nifedipine and nimodipine; class 2 are the relatively hydrophilic bases such as verapamil and diltiazem; class 3 are the diphenylalkylamines such as flunarizine. Representatives from all three classes have been found useful in migraine prophylaxis (Tables 3 and 4), and the characteristics of the clinical response, in part, reflect these differences.

The overall clinical response to these agents as a group compares favorably with, and may even exceed, the responses obtained with other prophylactic regimes (Table 3). Side effect potential is similarly no worse than that of existing therapies (88). Despite an early report that <u>severity</u> of attacks was not affected by treatment with flunarizine (4,71), subsequent studies with flunarizine (73), nifedipine (59), nimodipine (46) and verapamil (105) indicate that both the frequency <u>and</u> severity of attacks are reduced. Calcium antagonists seem to be equally effective against attacks of both common and classical migraine (71,73,76,105).

TABLE 4.   <u>Subclassification of Calcium Antagonists</u>
       <u>And Studies Reporting Their Antimigraine Actions:</u>
   (Classification according to Spedding, Reference 106)

<u>Class 1:</u>
       Dihydropyridines:
             Nifedipine   Data Source a
             Nimodipine   Data Source b

<u>Class 2:</u>
       Hydrophilic bases:
             Verapamil   Data Source c

<u>Class 3.:</u>
       Diphenylalkalamines:
             Flunarizine   Data Source d

Data Source = reference numbers:
a = Reference 59.
b = References 46, 52, and 76.
c = References 74 and 105.
d = References 28, 31, 44, 71, 73, and 134.

There are important differences between these agents when time to onset of anti-migraine effects is considered. The beneficial effects of flunarizine, for instance, develop over 3-4 months of treatment (4,5,44,73). Similarly, the time-lag before efficacy as seen with nimodipine is 2-4 weeks (46,76). In marked contrast, the effects of verapamil appear to be rapid in onset (105). Despite its slow onset of action, flunarizine has the important practical advantage in that it can be given in a single daily dose.

The calcium antagonists have been suggested to be of benefit in migraine because they inhibit intracerebral vasoconstriction irrespective of the initiating stimulus (76,90,91), but a number of observations are difficult to reconcile with this interpretation. Thus, calcium antagonists are effective against common migraine when cerebral blood flow studies show no significant reduction in blood flow at any time (82). Moreover, although in classical migraine a gradually spreading reduction in cerebral blood flow is observed, this is not considered to result from vasospasm (83). Similarly, the delay in onset of action of certain of these drugs is difficult to reconcile with an effect to inhibit vasospasm since prominent vascular relaxant effects are evident within minutes of drug administration (100). Finally, in this context, the effect of flunarizine deserves comment. Flunarizine is more than 10,000 times less active than nimodipine in inhibiting contraction of canine basilar artery in vitro (91) and, according to the hypothesis, ought to be significantly less active in migraine. In fact, the daily dose of flunarizine used to obtain a broadly similar anti-migraine response (Table 3) is, at 10 mg, some 12 times less than that of nimodipine, namely 120 mg (46,76). The discrepancy is too great for pharmacokinetic factors to be the explanation and reveals a major flaw in the attempt to link in vitro vasodilator potency of these agents with in vivo efficacy in migraine (91).

Clearly, the mode of action of calcium antagonists is more complex than a simple effect to relax vasospasm. Indeed, it would be naive to suppose that any single action could explain the effect of such a disparate group of compounds in so complex a condition. In seeking alternative explanations, there is no lack of possibilities since few physiological processes can function for long in the absence of calcium. Bearing on the theme developed earlier, it is possible that the calcium antagonists could interfere with the development of the proposed "sterile" inflammatory response of migraine. For instance, activation of phospholipase A_2 by a variety of stimuli follows an increased calcium flux into the membrane (132) and the process can be inhibited both by the absence of extracellular calcium and by calcium antagonists (8).

THERAPIES OF THE FUTURE

In attempting to see what the future might hold for the therapy of migraine, two developments, although very much at the preliminary stage, show signs of promise and, perhaps most encouragingly, introduce novel concepts into the therapy of migraine. The first is the use of domperidone in "complete" migraine. The second is the demonstration that MDL 72222, a selective antagonist at 5-HT neuronal receptors, is effective as symptomatic treatment.

Domperidone in "complete" migraine:

Domperidone is a dopamine D_2 receptor antagonist with both anti-emetic and gastrokinetic properties (21). Given intravenously during attacks, the compound relieves the symptoms of nausea and vomiting (55). In a double-blind, placebo-controlled, crossover study in 19 patients, Waelkens (124) reported that a single high dose of domperidone (30 mg), given orally up to 48h before an attack, prevented 60% of attacks developing. The patients were pre-selected to include only those in whom consistent physical and psychic signs warned of an impending attack; these patients suffer from "complete" migraine as defined by Blau (16). In a follow-up publication (125), the effect of domperidone was shown to be dose-related over the range 20, 30, and 40 mg, and to be critically dependent on the length of time before the anticipated attack that treatment was given. In general, the longer the pretreatment time the better the response; treatments within 6h of an attack were generally ineffective (125).

At this stage, there is no satisfactory explanation for this remarkable phenomenon which falls somewhere between the prophylactic approach and symptomatic treatment. It implies that in certain patients physiological events occur many hours before the full-blown attack develops which are critical to its genesis; perhaps most encouragingly these events are susceptible to pharmacological intervention. The pharmacological effects of domperidone have been extensively evaluated (21). What is particularly needed now is a thorough study of patients with "complete" migraine during the day prior to the attack. Establishment of the mechanism of the unique type of pharmacological intervention represented by domperidone in "complete" migraine might furnish leads to the development of novel therapies for the vast majority of migraine patients in whom advance warning of an attack is rarely given.

Symptomatic treatment with MDL 72222, a selective inhibitor of neuronal 5-HT receptors:

Since Sicuteri in 1959 introduced methysergide into prophylaxis on the basis of its potent 5-HT receptor antagonist activity, convincing biochemical, pharmacological, and anatomical evidence has accumulated ensuring that 5-HT has retained its place as the naturally-occurring substance with the strongest claim for a role in the pathophysiology of migraine (9,10,25,37,38,42). In man, 5-HT causes pain both by a direct action (47,61) and by sensitizing the sensory afferent fibers to other nociceptive stimuli (17,102). Specific 5-HT receptors, quite distinct from the $5-HT_2$ receptors thought to play a role in the prophylactic effects of agents such as methysergide and pizotifen, mediate the afferent neuronal stimulant effects of 5-HT (40). On the basis of a hypothesis implicating 5-HT in the pain production of the acute attack (39), a compound with potent and selective blocking activity at sensory neuronal 5-HT receptors, MDL 72222 (1alphaH, 5alphaH tropan-3alpha-yl

3,5-dichlorobenzoate), has recently been developed (41) and evaluated as symptomatic treatment. Under both open (43) and double-blind, placebo-controlled (70) conditions MDL 72222 (10-40 mg administered intravenously) proved an effective and well-tolerated treatment for the acute attack.

This encouraging clinical response seems likely to result from blockade of neuronal 5-HT receptors by MDL 72222. Firstly, the doses of MDL 72222 used are similar to those which in animal experiments produce highly selective blockade of afferent neuronal 5-HT receptors (41). Secondly, in a double-blind, placebo-controlled, crossover study in normal volunteers, a dose of 5-HT which was beneficial in migraine (20 mg, intravenously) markedly attenuated the flare response to intradermally injected 5-HT (Orwin and Fozard, unpublished observations) providing direct evidence that blockade of afferent neuronal 5-HT receptors is obtained in man. Finally, MDL 72222 does not have any of the properties of those agents used routinely in the treatment of the acute attack; even in high doses, the compound is neither analgesic nor anti-inflammatory, has no dopamine, histamine or muscarine receptor blocking properties which might bestow anti-emetic activity, and is not a vasoconstrictor (41,54).

These studies with MDL 72222 indicate that rapid, safe, and effective symptomatic treatment of migraine can be achieved by a novel mechanism. Other compounds which, like MDL 72222, cause selective blockade of excitatory neuronal 5-HT receptors have been described (29,30) and it seems certain that this new approach to treatment will be the subject of considerable clinical interest in the immediate future.

CONCLUSION

This critique of the principal therapies for migraine reveals a situation which falls well short of ideal; in effect, there exist no truly satisfactory prophylactic or symptomatic treatments. There are, nevertheless, signs of progress: certain calcium antagonists, despite being in the very early stages of clinical evaluation, show exciting promise in prophylaxis; single dose domperidone in the premonitory stages of an attack, and MDL 72222, an antagonist at 5-HT neuronal receptors, illustrate radical and potentially exciting new approaches to symptomatic treatment. Further progress will come most speedily from further elucidation of etiology by innovative clinical investigators using the very latest technologies; it will also come from the careful analysis of the actions of drugs used in, and developed for, the condition. In terms of the introductory analogy, the goal must be to bring the target(s) for the therapeutic bullets of the future increasingly into view. Only then will a rational approach to drug development be possible and the clinician be provided with the means whereby the therapeutic target can be consistently struck.

REFERENCES

1. Ala-Hurula, V. (1982): Eur. J. Clin. Pharmac., 21:397.
2. Ala-Hurula, V., Myllylä, V. V., Arvela, P., Heikkilä, J., Kärki, N., and Hokkanen, E. (1979): Eur. J. Clin. Pharmac., 15:51.
3. Amery, W. K. (1982): Cephalagia, 2:83.
4. Amery, W. K. (1983): Headache, 23:70.
5. Amery, W. K., Caers, L. I., and Aerts, T. J. L. (1985): Headache, 25:249.
6. Amery, W. K., Wauquier, A., Van Nueten, J. M., De Clerck, F., Van Reempts, J. V., and Janssen, P. A. J. (1981): Drugs Exp. Clin. Res., 7:1.
7. Andersson, P. G., Dahl, S., Hansen, J. H., Hedman, C., Kristensen, T. N., and de Fine Olivarius, B. (1983): Cephalagia, 3:207.
8. Ansiello, D. A., and Zusman, R. M. (1984): Biochem. J., 220:139.
9. Anthony, M., Hinterberger, H., and Lance, J. W. (1969): Res. Clin. Stud. Headache, 2:29.
10. Anthony, M., and Lance, J. W. (1975): In: Modern Topics in Migraine, edited by J. Pearce, pp. 107-113. Heinemann, London.
11. Apesos, J., and Folse, R. (1979): Arch. Surg., 114:964.
12. Baumrucker, J. F. (1973): N. Engl. J. Med., 288:916.
13. Behan, P. O., and Reid, M. (1980): Practitioner, 224:201.
14. Benedict, C. R., and Robertson, D. (1979): Amer. J. Med., 67:177.
15. Berde, B., Cerletti, A., Dengler, H. J., and Zoglio, M. A. (1970): In: Background to Migraine, Volume 3, edited by A. L. A. Cochrane, pp. 80-102. Heinemann, London.
16. Blau, J. N. (1980): Brit. Med. J., 2:658.
17. Bleehen, T., and Keele, C. A. (1977): Pain, 3:367.
18. Blundell, J. E. (1977): Int. J. Obesity, 1:15.
19. Bradfield, J. M. (1976): Drugs, 12:449.
20. Briggs, R. S., and Millac, P. A. (1979): Headache, 19:379.
21. Brogden, R. N., Carmine, A. A., Heel, R. C., Speight, T. M., and Avery, G. S. (1982): Drugs, 24:360.
22. Campbell, W. B., Johnson, A. R., Callahan, K. S., and Graham, R. M. (1981): Lancet, 2:1382.
23. Clineschmidt, B. V., and Bunting, P. R. (1980): Prog. Neuro-Psychopharmacol., 4:327.
24. Cohen, M. L., Fuller, R. W., and Kurz, K. D. (1983): J. Pharmacol. Exp. Ther., 227:327.
25. Crook, M. (1981): Biochem. Soc. Trans., 9:351.
26. Crooks, J., Stephen, S. A., and Brass, W. (1964): Brit. Med. J., 1:221.
27. Dalessio, D. J. (1978): Med. Clin. North America, 62:429.
28. Diamond, S., and Schenbaum, H. (1983): Headache, 23:39.
29. Donatsch, P., Engel, G., Richardson, B. P., and Stadler, P. A. (1984): Brit. J. Pharmac., 81:34P.

30. Donatsch, P., Engel, G., Richardson, B. P., and Stadler, P. A. (1984): Brit. J. Pharmac., 81:35P.
31. Drillisch, C., and Girke, W. (1980): Med. Welt., 31:1870.
32. Drugs and Therapeutic Bulletin (1964): 2:57.
33. Enna, S. J., and Kendall, D. A. (1981): J. Clin. Psychopharmacol., 1:12S.
34. Featherstone, H. J. (1983): West. J. Med., 138:416.
35. Flower, R. J. (1974): Pharmacol. Rev., 26:33.
36. Forssman, B., Lindblad, C. J., and Zbornikova, V. (1983): Headache, 23:188-190.
37. Fozard, J. R. (1975): J. Pharm. Pharmacol., 27:297.
38. Fozard, J. R. (1982): In: Drugs and Platelets, Progress in Pharmacology, Volume 4, edited by P. A. Van Zwieten and E. Schönbaum, pp. 135-146. Fischer, Stuttgart.
39. Fozard, J. R. (1982): In: Headache: Physiopathological and Clinical Concepts, Advances in Neurology, Volume 33, edited by M. Critchley, A. P. Friedman, S. Gorini, and F. Sicuteri, pp. 295-307. Raven Press, New York.
40. Fozard, J. R. (1984): Neuropharmacology, 23:1473.
41. Fozard, J. R. (1984): Naunyn-Schmiedeberg's Arch. Pharmac., 326:36.
42. Fozard, J. R. (1985): In: Vascular Neuroeffector Mechanisms. edited by J. A. Bevan, T. Godfraind, R. A. Maxwell, J. C. Stodet, and M. Worcel, pp. 321-328. Elsevier, Amsterdam.
43. Fozard, J. R., Loisy, C., and Tell, G. (1985): In: Advances in Migraine Research, edited by F. C. Rose. Karger, Basel.
44. Frenken, C. W. G. M., and Niujten, S. T. M. (1984): Clin. Neurol. Neurosurg., 86:17.
45. Gaddum, J. H., and Picarelli, Z. P. (1957): Brit. J. Pharmac., 12:323.
46. Gelmers, H. J. (1983): Headache, 23:106.
47. Greaves, M. W., and Schuster, S. (1967): J. Physiol. (Lond.), 193:255.
48. Hakkarainen, H., and Allonen, H. (1982): Headache, 22:10.
49. Hakkarainen, H., Gustafsson, B. and Stockman, O. (1978): Headache, 18:35.
50. Hakkarainen, H., Vapaatalo, H., Gothoni, G., and Parantainen, J. (1979): Lancet, 2:326.
51. Harrington, R. A., Hamilton, C. W., Brogden, R. N., Linkewich, J. A., Romankiewicz, J. A., and Heel, R. C. (1983): Drugs, 25:451.
52. Havanka-Kanniainen, H., Myllylä, V., and Hokkanen, E. (1982): Acta Neurol. Scandinav., 90:77 (Suppl.)
53. Ibraheem, J. J., Paalzow, L., and Tfelt-Hansen, P. (1982): Eur. J. Clin. Pharmac., 23:235.
54. Investigational Brochure (1984): MDL 72222. Merrell-Dow Research Institute, Strasbourg, France.
55. Jaecques, N., Lambrecht, A., Schietterkatte, L., and Waelkens, J. (1979): Postgrad. Med. J., 55:51 (Suppl. 1).

56. Janssen, P. A. J. (1983): Trends Pharmacol. Sci., 4:198.
57. Janssen, P. A. J. (1983): Trends Pharmacol. Sci., 4:412.
58. Joyce, D. A., and Gubbay, S. S. (1982): Brit. Med. J., 285:260.
59. Kahen, A., Weber, S., Amor, B., Guerin, F., and Degeorges, M. (1983): N. Engl. J. Med., 308:1102.
60. Kangasniemi, P., and Hedman, C. (1984): Cephalagia, 4:91.
61. Keele, C. A., and Armstrong, D. (1964): Substances Producing Pain and Itch. Williams & Wilkins Company, Baltimore.
62. Kreel, L. (1969): Arch. Gastroenterol., 6:155.
63. Kudrow, L. (1978): Psychosomatics, 19:685-687; 691-693.
64. Kuehl, F. A., and Egan, R. W. (1980): Science, 210:978.
65. Lance, J. W. (1982): Mechanism and Management of Headache, 4th Edition. Butterworths, London.
66. Lance, J. W., and Anthony, M. (1966): Arch. Neurol., 15:356.
67. Lance, J. W., Anthony, M., and Somerville, B. (1970): Brit. Med. J., 2:327.
68. Lauritzen, M., and Olesen, J. (1984): Brain; 107:447.
69. Leysen, J. E., Awouters, F., Kennis, L., Laduron, P. M., Vandenberk, J., and Janssen, P. A. J. (1981): Life Sci., 28:1015.
70. Loisy, C., Beorchia, S., Centonze, V., Fozard, J. R., Schechter, P. J., and Tell, G. P. (1985): Cephalagia, 5:79.
71. Louis, P. (1981): Headache, 21:235.
72. Louis, P. (1985): Cephalagia, (in press)
73. Louis, P., and Spierings, E. L. H. (1982): Cephalagia, 2:197.
74. Markley, H. G., Cheronis, J. C. D., and Peipho, R. W. (1983): Neurology, 33:175 (Suppl.).
75. Medical Letter (1979): 21:77-78.
76. Meyer, J. S., and Hardenberg, J. (1983): Headache, 23:266.
77. Mikkelsen, E., Pedersen, O. L., Ostergaard, J. R., and Pedersen, S. E. (1981): Arch. Int. Pharmacodyn., 252:241.
78. Moskowitz, M. A. (1984): Ann. Neurol., 16:157.
79. Müller-Schweinitzer, E. (1976): Naunyn-Schmiedeberg's Arch. Pharmacol., 295:41.
80. Mylecharane, E. J., Spira, P. J., Misbach, J., Duckworth, J. W., and Lance, J. W. (1978): Eur. J. Pharmac., 48:1.
81. Olesen, J. (1978): Headache, 18:268.
82. Olesen, J., Larsen, B., and Lauritzen, M. (1981): Ann. Neurol., 9:344.
83. Olesen, J., and Lauritzen, M. (1984): In: The Pharmacological Basis of Migraine Therapy, edited by W. K. Amery, J. M. Van Nueten, and A. Wauquier, pp. 7-18. Pitman, London.
84. Olesen, J., Tfelt-Hansen, P., Henriksen, L., and Larsen, B. (1981): Lancet, 2:438.

85. Orton, D. A., and Richardson, R. J. (1982): Postgrad. Med. J., 58:6.
86. Ostergaard, J. R., Mikkelsen, E., and Vodby, B. (1981): Cephalagia, 1:223.
87. Peatfield, R. (1983): Drugs, 26:364.
88. Peatfield, R. C., Fozard, J. R., and Rose, F. C. (1985): In: Handbook of Clinical Neurology, Volume 4, edited by F. C. Rose. Elsevier, Amsterdam.
89. Peatfield, R. C., Petty, R. G., and Rose, F. C. (1983): Cephalagia, 3:129.
90. Peroutka, S. J. (1983): Headache, 23:278.
91. Peroutka, S. J., Banghart, S. B., and Allen, G. S. (1984): Headache, 24:55.
92. Peroutka, S. J., and Snyder, S. H. (1979): Molec. Pharmac., 16:687.
93. Peroutka, S. J., and Snyder, S. H. (1980): Science, 210:88.
94. Rabkin, R., Stables, D. P., Levin, N. W., and Suzman, M. M. (1966): Amer. J. Cardiol., 18:370.
95. Ross-Lee, L. M., Eadie, M. J., Heazlewood, V., Bochner, F., and Tyrer, J. H. (1983): Eur. J. Clin. Pharmac., 24:777.
96. Sanger, G. (1985): In: Mechanisms of Gastrointestinal Motility and Secretion, edited by A. Bennett, and G. Velo. Plenum Press, New York.
97. Saper, J. R. (1978): JAMA, 239:2480.
98. Saxena, P. R., and De Vlaam-Schluter, G. M. (1974): Headache, 13:142.
99. Schulze-Delrieu, K. (1981): N. Engl. J. Med., 305:28.
100. Schwartz, M. L., Rotmensch, H. H., Vlasses, P. H., and Ferguson, R. K. (1984): Arch. Intern. Med., 144:1425.
101. Shanks, R. G. (1985): In: Proc. Astra Symposium "Migraine and Beta-Blockade", Munich, May, 1984.
102. Sicuteri, F., Fanciullacci, M., Franchi, G., and Del Bianco, P. L. (1965): Life Sci., 4:309.
103. Simon, L. S., and Mills, J. A. (1980): New Engl. J. Med., 302:1179-1185; 1237-1243.
104. Slettnes, O., and Sjaastad, O. (1977): In: Headache: New Vistas, edited by F. Sicuteri, pp. 201-204. Biomedical Press, Florence.
105. Solomon, G. D., Steel, J. G., and Spaccavento, L. J. (1983): JAMA, 250:2500.
106. Spedding, M. (1985): Trends Pharmacol. Sci., 6:109.
107. Spira, P. J., Mylecharane, E. J., and Lance, J. W. (1976): Res. Clin. Stud. Headache, 4:37.
108. Stellar, S., Ahrens, S. P., Meibohm, A. R., and Reines, S. A. (1984): JAMA, 252:2576.
109. Stensrud, P., and Sjaastad, O. (1980): Headache, 20:204.
110. Tfelt-Hansen, P., Eickhoff, J. H., and Olesen, J. (1980): Acta Pharmacol. Toxicol., 47:151.
111. Tfelt-Hansen, P., and Olesen, J. (1980): Eur. Neurol., 19:163.
112. Tfelt-Hansen, P., and Olesen, J. (1984): Cephalagia, 4:107.

113. Tfelt-Hansen, P., Olesen, J., Aebelholt-Krabbe, A., Melgaard, B., and Veilis, B. (1980): J. Neurol. Neurosurg. Psychiat., 43:369.
114. Tfelt-Hansen, P., Paalzow, L., and Ibraheem, J. J. (1982): Brit. J. Clin. Pharmac., 13:239.
115. Tfelt-Hansen, P., Standnes, B., Kangasniemi, P., Hakkarainen, H., and Olesen, J. (1984): Acta Neurol. Scandinav., 69:1.
116. Tokola, R., and Hokkanen, E. (1978): Brit. Med. J., 2:1089.
117. Tokola, R. A., and Neuvonen, P. J. (1981): Acta Pharmacol. Toxicol., 49:78 (Suppl. 1).
118. Tokola, R. A., and Neuvonen, P. J. (1984): Brit. J. Clin. Pharmac., 17:67.
119. Venter, C. P., Joubert, P. H., and Buys, A. C. (1984): Brit. Med. J., 289:288.
120. Vilming, S., Standnes, B., and Hedman, C. (1985): Cephalagia, 5:17.
121. Volans, G. N. (1974): Brit. Med. J., 4:265.
122. Volans, G. N. (1975): Brit. J. Clin. Pharmac., 2:57.
123. Volans, G. N. (1978): Clin. Pharmacokinetics, 3:313.
124. Waelkens, J. (1982): Brit. Med. J., 284:944.
125. Waelkens, J. (1984): Cephalagia, 4:85.
126. Wainscott, G., Kaspi, T., and Volans, G. N. (1976): Brit. J. Clin. Pharmac., 3:1015.
127. Waters, W. E. (1970): Brit. Med. J., 2:325.
128. Weerasuriya, K., Patel, L., and Turner, P. (1982): Cephalagia, 2:33.
129. Weksler, B. B., Gillick, M., and Pink, J. (1977): Blood, 49:185.
130. Wilkinson, M. (1983): Cephalagia, 3:61.
131. Wilkinson, M., Williams, K., and Leyton, M. (1978): Res. Clin. Stud. Headache, 6:141.
132. Withnall, M. T., Brown, T. J., and Diocee, B. K. (1984): Biochem. Biophys. Res. Comm., 121:507.
133. Wolff, H. G. (1963): Headache and Other Head Pain, 2nd Edition. Oxford University Press, New York.
134. Wörz, R., and Drillisch, C. (1983): Munch. Med. Wschr., 125:711.
135. Wykes, P. (1968): Practitioner, 200:702.
136. Yamamoto, M., and Meyer, J. S. (1980): Headache, 20:321.

The Management of Headache, edited by F. Clifford Rose. Raven Press, New York © 1988.

CLUSTER HEADACHE

J. Keith Campbell, MD, FRCP (Edin)

Department of Neurology, Mayo Clinic, 200 First Street, S. W., Rochester, Minnesota 55905, U.S.A.

Among the many painful conditions that affect the head, the one known by the most names is also unique in several other respects. Cluster headache, Horton's headache, histaminic cephalgia, or migrainous neuralgia, as the condition is variously known, is without doubt the most painful recurrent headache and the one that produces the most stereotyped attacks, both in the individual patient and in fellow sufferers. Despite its readily recognizable features, the syndrome continues to be misdiagnosed as trigeminal neuralgia, sinus or dental disease, and is therefore ineffectually treated -- an unfortunate circumstance because correct diagnosis can lead to successful management in most patients. Although the condition has been partially described previously (17), Horton (19,21) and subsequently Symonds (41) fully delineated its clinical features and proposed several treatments, including the use of ergotamine tartrate. Horton believed histamine was involved in the production of the pain and championed histamine desensitization as an effective therapy for many years (20). The name "histaminic cephalgia" has gradually been displaced in favor of the term used by Kunkle et al. (28), "cluster headache," which accurately characterizes the periodicity of the condition in many patients.

Classification and Terminology

In episodic cluster headache, attacks of pain occur daily for days, weeks or months before an attack-free period of remission occurs. This respite may last from weeks to years before another cluster (of attacks) develops. In chronic cluster headache, attacks of pain occur at least twice per week for more than two years without a remission (11). This chronic phase of the disease may develop de novo or it may follow a period of episodic cluster headache. Chronic cluster headache can, therefore, be divided into primary and secondary chronic types. Approximately 10-15% of patients with this disorder have one of the chronic varieties.

Incidence, Sex Ratio, and Family History

Compared with tension headache or migraine, cluster headache is uncommon. In many headache clinic populations, migraine is ten to fifty times more common than cluster headache. In the general population, the comparative percentages vary because many migraine sufferers do not seek help, whereas the intensity of cluster headache can rarely be endured in silence. It is predominantly a disease of males; the male to female ratio being at least 5:1 and probably higher. Inheritance does not seem to be a factor, as a positive family history of cluster headache is rarely found (11). The incidence of migraine in patients with cluster headache is no higher than in the general population. For this and other reasons, migraine and cluster headache are most likely not related, apart from the belief that both are due to vasodilatation.

CLINICAL FEATURES

Attacks often begin in the late twenties, but onset has been described as early as three years of age or as late as the seventh decade. In most patients, the first cluster of attacks persists from two to six weeks and is followed by a period of freedom lasting months or even years. With time, however, the clusters become seasonal and then more frequent and longer lasting. During a cluster, the patient may experience from one to three or more attacks per 24 hours, and the episodes commonly occur at similar times throughout the 24 hours for many days. Onset during the night, or one to two hours after going to sleep is common. This time may correspond to the onset of rapid eye movement sleep and can result in deprivation of sleep in chronic sufferers, particularly when they avoid sleep for fear of inducing a further attack. With increasing age, the distinct clustering pattern may be less recognizable; in a high percentage of patients, periods of relief become less common, and the condition enters the chronic phase in which attacks may occur daily for months or years. In these patients, the condition may persist into old age but, in many, the attacks eventually cease. No ethnic group appears immune to the development of the syndrome.

The Acute Attack

Whether the patient is in the episodic phase or the chronic phase, the attacks of pain are identical for any individual. The pain is strictly unilateral and almost always remains on the same side of the head; rarely, it may switch to the opposite side in a subsequent cluster. The pain is generally felt in the retro-orbital and temporal region but may be maximal in the cheek or jaw (lower-half headache) (14). It is usually described as steady or boring and of terrible intensity ("suicide headache"). Graphic descriptions of the "eye being pushed out" or "an auger going through the eye" are very common. Onset is usually abrupt or preceded by a brief sensation of pressure in the soon-to-be-painful area. The pain intensifies very rapidly, peaking in 5-10 minutes and then persisting for 45 minutes to two hours. Toward the end of this time, brief periods of slight relief are followed by several transient peaks of pain before the attack subsides over a few minutes. Occasional attacks last twice as long. The patient is then completely free from pain, but exhausted; however, the respite may be short-lived because another attack may occur shortly, especially if the subject falls asleep. During the pain, the subject is almost invariably unwilling to lie down as this increases the intensity; unlike patients with migraine, they are restless and prefer to pace about or sit during an attack. Others will adopt unusual postures during the pain such as lying prone on the bed with their head hung down to the floor. Yet others will remain outside, even in freezing weather, for the duration of the attack. An otherwise rational person may strike his head against a wall or hurt himself in another way as a distraction from the anguish suffered during an attack of cluster headache. Most patients prefer to be alone during the attack, possibly to withdraw from distressed relatives who are unable to give comfort to the sufferer. Some will apply ice to the painful region, others prefer hot applications; almost all will press on the scalp or the eye to try to obtain relief. During the pain, many patients consider suicide, but very few attempt it. Even watching a patient during an attack of cluster headache is a harrowing experience.

Associated Features

During the pain of cluster headache, which is believed to be due to extracranial and possibly intracranial vasodilatation, the nose on the side of the pain is generally blocked; this factor in turn leads to ipsilateral overflow of tears caused by blockage of the nasolacrimal duct. The conjunctiva is injected ipsilaterally and the superficial temporal artery may be visibly distended. Sweating and facial flushing on the side of the pain have been described but are rare. Nasal drainage usually signals the end of the attack. Ptosis and miosis on the side of the pain are common. This partial Horner's syndrome may persist between the attacks after a cluster has been present for some weeks and is believed to be due to compression of the sympathetic plexus secondary to vasodilatation in the region of the carotid siphon. Facial sweating is always preserved.

Patients who have cluster headaches have a high incidence of duodenal ulceration and elevated gastric acid levels that may approach those seen in the Zollinger-Ellison syndrome. It is also claimed they have coarse facial skin of the peau d'orange type, deep nasolabial folds, and an increased incidence of hazel eye color (25). Many of the patients are heavy cigarette smokers and tend to drink more alcohol than control subjects.

Photophobia during the painful stage is less common than in migraine, but may occur and be accompanied by sonophobia. Nausea during the attack is uncommon and often times due to analgesic or ergotamine usage. Facial swelling, most often periorbital in location, may develop with repeated attacks. Infrequently, transient localized swellings of the palate, ipsilateral to the pain can be observed. More commonly, the patient may complain that the palate feels swollen, but no abnormality can be detected by the examiner, even during an attack.

An observation, so far unexplained, is that during the active headache phase in male patients, the plasma testosterone is significantly lower than values in control patients or in the subjects during periods of remission (23,33). More recently, it has been suggested that the lowered testosterone level may be secondary to disordered sleep patterns during the active headache period (37).

PATHOPHYSIOLOGY

The vascular changes during an attack are difficult to study and reported findings are conflicting. Although vasodilatation is generally believed to be responsible for the pain, the site of this increased flow is not fully known. Several studies suggested dilatation of the ophthalmic and internal carotid arteries (4,13), whereas a radiographic study showed constriction of the carotid siphon during an attack (13). Blood flow studies (38) showed increased hemispheric flow bilaterally during a headache, with the greatest flow contralateral to the pain. A tomographic blood flow study by Olesen and his co-workers (22) also failed to show evidence that regional cerebral blood flow changed to any appreciable extent during the painful attack. The small increases in blood flow observed were thought to be due to pain activation of receptor neurons rather than a primary event. Thermographic studies (16,26) have shown persistent cold spots in the forehead ipsilateral to the pain in the distribution of the supraorbital artery, a terminal branch of the ophthalmic artery.

The belief that vasodilatation causes the pain is supported by the observation that various vasodilators will precipitate an attack within a few minutes when the patient is in the clustering phase. Nitroglycerine (1 mg sublingually), histamine (0.35 mg intravenously or subcutaneously), and alcohol perorally are all effective. Most patients discover very quickly that they cannot drink alcohol in any form as soon as a cluster develops, but, once a period of remission is entered, alcohol usually fails to precipitate an attack. Other evidence for vasodilatation causing the pain comes from the fact that drugs that produce vasoconstriction such as norepinephrine, ergotamine tartrate, and dihydroergotamine mesylate will give relief rapidly when administered by an appropriate route.

The pathogenesis of cluster headache is unknown. Several interesting observations suggest that histamine may have a role in the cause of the condition. During painful attacks, increased histamine levels in the blood and urine have been detected (1,40), but whether this is a primary or secondary phenomenon is unknown. Morphologic studies on the increased number (29,36) and abnormal distribution (3) of mast cells in the forehead skin of patients with cluster headache support the theory that local release of histamine is involved in some way in this condition. Evidence to the contrary, however, comes from the observations that blockage of both H_1 and H_2 histamine receptors by antihistamine drugs has no effect on the painful attacks (2,8). Allergic phenomena and dietary factors seem to be unimportant in cluster headache. Few psychologic factors seem to be operative in this condition, although many of the patients are of the hard-driving executive type. Unlike migraineurs, patients with cluster headache rarely become addicted to drugs and seldom develop pain behavior traits.

Differential Diagnosis

The diagnosis of cluster headache is essentially clinical and depends upon obtaining an accurate history from the patient. Confirmation of the periodicity, rapidity of onset and resolution, presence of conjunctival injection, ptosis and altered behavior during the attack from the spouse or relatives is helpful. Despite the stereotyped nature of the attacks from episode to episode and from patient to patient, the diagnosis is often missed for several years. Conditions which cause episodic, unilateral head and face pain should be considered, but should be easy to exclude. Trigeminal neuralgia, sinusitis, dental disease and glaucoma may superficially mimic the pain of cluster headache, but in each the temporal profile, lack of associated autonomic features and past history should allow easy differentiation. Similarly, migraine, temporal arteritis, and the headache of intracranial space-occupying lesions should give little cause for difficulty in reaching a diagnosis of cluster headache. Episodic headache due to pheochromocytoma or hypoglycemia produced by endogenous or exogenous excess insulin is likely to be bilateral and unaccompanied by tearing, nasal stuffiness or ptosis and is rarely so dramatic in onset or resolution. Orbital, retro-orbital and frontal pain, associated with an incomplete Horner's syndrome, can result from ipsilateral dissection of the carotid artery (15,32) but, unlike the pain of cluster headache, it is not episodic and does not produce the restlessness so characteristic of this condition. The pain of a carotid dissection generally persists from days to months. The pain associated with the Tolosa-Hunt syndrome and Raeder's paratrigeminal syndrome are accompanied by oculomotor or trigeminal nerve dysfunction which should easily prevent confusion with cluster headache. Similarly, compression of the third nerve by an aneurysm should be easy to distinguish from cluster pain, especially when a partial or complete third nerve palsy is detected.

Investigations

In most patients, the diagnosis is so certain on clinical grounds that special neurologic investigations are unnecessary. As part of the management, however, it may be advisable to obtain a contrast-enhanced computed tomogram (CT scan) to help to reassure the patients and their relatives that the extremely painful attacks are not due to major intracranial pathology. The CT scan should detect those conditions such as a pituitary tumor or an arteriovenous malformation which have been shown in single case reports to mimic cluster headache. Examination of the eyes should include measurement of the ocular tension to detect glaucoma. Tests of a general nature are needed to determine any contraindications to the use of various medications.

MANAGEMENT

The patient and relatives must be reassured that the sufferer is not alone and that the clinical pattern they describe is one that has been seen before. Care should be taken to reassure the patient that the syndrome, while unbearably painful, is benign and not life-threatening. Pain reduction but not cure should be promised. Many patients express relief when they realize they are not the only person ever to have suffered this painful condition.

Pharmacotherapy

The frequency, severity, and brevity of individual attacks of cluster headache and their lack of response to many symptomatic measures necessitate the use of a prophylactic program for most patients. The choice of preparation is determined by several factors such as the phase of the disorder (episodic or chronic) and by the presence or absence of other disease states such as hypertension and coronary or peripheral vascular insufficiency.

During the initial cluster or when the patient's past history suggests that a cluster will be of limited duration, relief can usually be obtained by administering a short course of corticosteroids. Several regimens have been shown effective --for example, 60 mg of prednisone as a single daily dose for 3 or 4 days, followed by a 10 mg reduction after every third or fourth day that thereby tapers the dose to zero over 18 or 24 days. Alternatively, an intramuscular injection of triamcinolone (Kenalog-40, 80 mg) or methylprednisolone (Depo-Medrol, 80-120 mg) can be employed to give a tapering corticosteroid blood level. Whichever program is used, the patient usually will obtain relief from the headaches until the lower dosages or blood levels of corticosteroids are approached. The course can be repeated several times, but thereafter the risk of side effects from these agents suggests that an alternative prophylactic program should be used if the cluster has not run its course. Ergotamine tartrate (1 or 2 mg) can be given orally or by rectal suppository on retiring to prevent nocturnal attacks of headache, but this may only postpone the attack until morning, when it may be more troublesome if it occurs when the patient is at work. Nevertheless, prophylactic use of ergotamine tartrate can be most valuable, but great care must be taken to regulate the dose if chronic ergotism is to be avoided. Most patients with cluster headache can be given 2 mg of ergotamine tartrate daily for several weeks without adverse effects. Nausea and peripheral paresthesias are common side effects of ergot regardless of the route of administration. Ergonovine maleate is a well tolerated ergot derivative which can be given in a dosage of 0.2 mg every 6 or 8 hours for prevention of headache. All ergot preparations are contra-indicated in pregnancy, in the presence of infection or known sensitivity to the drug.

Methysergide in a dosage range of 4-10 mg per day is effective in reducing or preventing cluster headache in about 60% of patients (24). The side effects, which include leg cramps, nausea and retention of fluid, are usually minor, and the drug seems better tolerated in these patients than in patients with migraine. The risk of retroperitoneal and other types of fibrosis is important only when methysergide must be taken for months or longer. For the episodic phase of cluster headache, this drug may be needed for only a few weeks, so that the risk of serious side effects is low. If methysergide gives relief, the lowest effective dose should be determined and the preparation continued for two to four weeks after the last attack. It can be restarted if the headaches return after discontinuation of the drug. If the cluster is very long or if the patient has gone into the chronic phase of the disorder, methysergide can be taken for up to six months, at which time it must be discontinued for at least four weeks while an intravenous pyelogram, serum creatinine level and chest roentgenogram are obtained. If the patient has no signs of fibrosis, treatment with methysergide can be continued for a further three to six months, after which the fibrotic complications should again be sought.

For patients in the chronic phase of cluster headache when attacks occur daily for years, relief may be obtained from lithium (12,24,30). Lithium carbonate, 300 mg three times daily, can be given initially and the dose adjusted at two weeks to obtain a serum lithium level of about 1.0 mEq/liter. Side effects at this level include a mild tremor of the limbs, gastrointestinal distress, and increased thirst. The therapeutic range is very narrow, and blood levels of more than 1.5 mEq/liter are to be avoided. Nephrotoxicity, goiter formation, and a permanent diabetes insipidus-like state have been reported after lithium treatment. In chronic cluster headache, lithium should have a beneficial effect within a week; however, the response may be delayed for several weeks. Although attacks may recur after some months, a renewed response to lithium may occur if the drug is withdrawn after a few weeks. In those patients who respond to lithium, the use of the drug should be discontinued every few months to determine whether the cluster headaches have subsided. While lithium is given, it is necessary to monitor the blood level at regular intervals to avoid the development of serious side effects. Thiazide diuretics should not be used concurrently as they can cause a rapid elevation of the blood levels to the toxic range.

Despite the treatments available, the management of patients with chronic cluster headache can be extremely difficult because many of them fail to respond, or respond only briefly to the programs already described. In such patients, a combination of several drugs may give relief. Methysergide and corticosteroids can be given together, or methysergide and lithium can be combined. Other combinations worth trying are corticosteroids and prophylactic ergot preparations. The latter can also be combined with methysergide as the drugs seem to act synergistically. When such potent agents are used, extreme care must be exercised to detect potentially serious side effects as soon as they occur. For many patients in the chronic phase, corticosteroids are the only preparations that give any relief. Side effects can be minimized by using the lowest effective dose, by using alternate-day dosage schedules, and by giving intermittent tapering courses with corticosteroid-free intervals. Despite these drastic measures, in some patients the chronic cluster headaches remain resistant to prophylactic measures. Other drugs that may be helpful in prophylaxis include chlorpromazine (7), indomethacin and cyproheptadine. Antihistamines of the H_1 and H_2 receptor blocking properties are of no value.

Symptomatic Treatment

Oral administration of drugs is generally ineffective in acute cluster headache because of the rapid onset and limited duration of the pain. The aerosol form of ergotamine tartrate may be helpful if the patient can use it correctly. Two inhalations deliver 0.72 mg of ergotamine tartrate, which should be taken at the onset of the pain. Lack of response to this mode of treatment is often due to failure to shake the canister to resuspend the drug or to incomplete inhalation (deep inspiration should be held for several seconds). Rectally administered ergotamine tartrate (1 or 2 mg) at the onset of an attack will often shorten the painful episode. Similarly, 2 mg ergotamine tartrate given sublingually may be useful. Dosage limitations must be stressed to minimize the risk of ergotism. Dihydroergotamine mesylate (DHE-45) 0.5 to 1 mg subcutaneously or intravenously, will often shorten an attack of cluster headache considerably. It is an inconvenient treatment for the sufferer whose attacks can occur at any time in the day, but those who have been instructed in self-administration often obtain good relief. Usually 2 to 4 mg/24 hours is well tolerated for several weeks. Unlike patients with migraine, those with cluster headache do not commonly develop ergot dependence or rebound headaches due to temporary reduction in ergot dosage. Analgesics are essentially useless in cluster headache because the intensity of the pain is such that only a narcotic would give relief and the recurrent nature of the attacks precludes the use of agents of this type.

Inhalation of oxygen via a loosely-applied face mask at a flow rate of 8-10 liters/minute can be dramatically effective in aborting a cluster headache (27). Oxygen is believed to help because of its vasoconstrictive properties. It is a harmless, but inconvenient therapy, requiring a bulky cylinder at home and at work if the patient has attacks both day and night.

Many other treatments have been proposed for chronic cluster headache. None have proven effective. Histamine desensitization (19,21), the administration of anticonvulsants, and estrogens are among those which have been abandoned. Currently being evaluated are the calcium channel antagonist class of drugs. Experience to date is too limited to draw any conclusions regarding their place in the treatment of cluster headache.

Surgical Treatment

Harris (18) and Dott (10) advocated injection of alcohol into the gasserian ganglion or trigeminal root section for the treatment of chronic migrainous neuralgia (cluster headache), but these procedures did not gain widespread acceptance and were gradually abandoned because of the high incidence of complications, including neuroparalytic keratitis, postoperative herpes keratitis, and anesthesia dolorosa of the denervated area. An occasional patient continued to have the pain of cluster headache, despite the procedure. Recently, however, interest has been renewed in the surgical relief of this condition. O'Brien and MacCabe (34) described three patients who had undergone selective trigeminal sensory rhizotomy via the posterior fossa and had experienced complete relief of intractable cluster headaches. The patients continued to have nasal stuffiness and corneal injection intermittently, but these episodes were painless. These results have been confirmed in three patients who were similarly treated by the author (5) and by a series of fifteen patients who have undergone percutaneous thermocoagulation of the gasserian ganglion with dramatic relief of symptoms in almost all patients (6). Transient weakness of the muscles of mastication on the side of the procedure is relatively common but rarely troublesome. Keratitis and anesthesia dolorosa are more serious complications of any destructive procedure on the trigeminal nerve. Maxwell (31) and

Watson (42) have both reported favorably on thermocoagulation of the gasserian ganglion for the treatment of cluster headache. Injection of glycerol into Meckle's cave has also been effective in producing pain relief in this condition (9).

CHRONIC PAROXYSMAL HEMICRANIA

This headache, which is probably a variety of cluster headache, was described by Sjaastad and Dale (39). The condition is seen most often in middle-aged women and is a severe paroxysmal hemicranial pain similar in intensity and location to cluster headache but differing in its short duration and high repetition rate. Attacks usually last ten to twenty minutes and may recur up to twelve times daily. Attacks tend to continue for months but, unlike true cluster headache, they are almost invariably terminated by small prophylactic doses of indomethacin. The course and natural history of this condition are unknown.

REFERENCES

1. Anthony, M., and Lance, J. W. (1971): Arch. Neurol., 25:225.
2. Anthony, M., Lord, G. D. A., and Lance, J. W. (1978): Headache, 18:261.
3. Appenzeller, O., Becker, W. J., and Ragaz, A. (1981): Arch. Neurol., 38:302.
4. Broch, A., Hørven, I., Nornes, H., Sjaastad, O., and Tønjum, A. (1970): Headache, 10:1.
5. Campbell, J. K. (1984): In: Cluster Headache, edited by N. T. Mathew, pp. 127–133. SP Medical and Scientific Books, New York.
6. Campbell, J. K., and Onofrio, B. M. Unpublished data.
7. Caviness, V. S., Jr., and O'Brien, P. (1980): Headache, 20:128.
8. Cuypers, J., Altenkirch, H., and Bunge, S. (1979): Eur. Neurol., 18:345.
9. Dalessio, D. J., Waltz, T., and Ott, K. (1984): Headache, 24:162.
10. Dott, N. M. (1951): Proc. R. Soc. Med., 44:1034.
11. Ekbom, K. (1970): Acta Neurol. Scandinav., 41.46:1–48, (Suppl.).
12. Ekbom, K. (1977): Headache, 17:39.
13. Ekbom, K., and Greitz, T. (1970): Acta Radiol. Diagn. (Stockh.), 10:177.
14. Ekbom, K., and Kugelberg, E. (1968): In: Brain and Mind Problems, pp. 482–489. Pensiero Science Publications, Rome.
15. Fisher, C. M. (1982): Headache, 22:60.
16. Friedman, A. P., and Wood, E. H. (1976): In: Medical Thermography, Theory and Clinical Applications, edited by S. Uematsu, pp. 80–84. Brentwood Publishing Corporation, Los Angeles.
17. Harris, W. (1926): Neuritis and Neuralgia, pp. 301–313. Oxford University Press, London.
18. Harris, W. (1936): Brit. Med. J., 1:457.
19. Horton, B. T. (1941): JAMA, 116:377.
20. Horton, B. T. (1961): Maryland State Med. J., 10:178.
21. Horton, B. T., MacLean, A. R., and Craig, W. M. (1939): Mayo Clin. Proc., 14:257.
22. Krabbe, A. A., Henriksen, L., and Olesen, J. (1984): Cephalagia, 4:17.
23. Kudrow, L. (1976): Headache, 16:28.
24. Kudrow, L. (1978): In: Current Concepts in Migraine Research, edited by R. Greene, pp. 159–163. Raven Press, New York.
25. Kudrow, L. (1979): Headache, 19:142.
26. Kudrow, L. (1979): Headache, 19:204.
27. Kudrow, L. (1981): Headache, 21:1.

28. Kunkle, E. C., Pfeiffer, J. B., Jr., Wilhoit, W. M., and
    Hamrick, L. W., Jr. (1952): Trans. Amer. Neurol.
    Assoc., 77:240.
29. Liberski, P. P., and Prusinski, A. (1982): Headache,
    22:115.
30. Manzoni, G. C., Bono, G., and Lafranchi, M., et al. (1983):
    Cephalagia, 3:109.
31. Maxwell, R. E. (1982): J. Neurosurg., 57:459.
32. Mokri, B., Sundt, T. M., Jr., and Houser, O. W. (1979):
    Arch. Neurol., 36:677.
33. Nelson, R. F. (1978): Headache, 18:265.
34. O'Brien, M. D., and MacCabe, J. J. (1981): In: Progress in
    Migraine Research, edited by F. C. Rose, and K. J.
    Zilkha, pp. 185-187. Pitman Books, Ltd., London.
35. Prusinski, A., and Liberski, P. P. (1979): Headache,
    19:102.
36. Romiti, A., Martelletti, P., Gallo, M. F., and Giacorazzo,
    M. (1983): Cephalagia, 3:41.
37. Sakai, F., and Meyer, J. S. (1978): Headache, 18:122.
38. Sjaastad, O., and Dale, I. (1976): Acta Neurol. Scandinav.,
    54:140.
39. Sjaastad, O., and Sjaastad, Ø. V. (1977): J. Neurol.,
    216:105.
40. Symonds, C. (1956): Brain, 79:217.
41. Watson, C. P., Morley, T. P., Richardson, J. C., Schutz,
    H., and Tasker, R. R. (1983): Headache, 23:289.

The Management of Headache, edited by F. Clifford Rose. Raven Press, New York © 1988.

MUSCLE CONTRACTION HEADACHE

Dewey K. Ziegler, MD

Chairman and Professor, Department of Neurology, University of Kansas College of Health Sciences and Hospital, 39th and Rainbow Boulevard, Kansas City, Kansas 66103, U.S.A.

History

It is interesting to begin the study of muscle contraction headache with a brief look at the history of the concept. Textbooks of neurology at the turn of the century contained descriptions of migraine that are much the same as those we use currently; for non-migrainous recurrent headache on the other hand, the discussion was different. In the text by Oppenheim (22), in 1900, for example, after a detailed discussion of migraine (included, interestingly enough, in the section on neuroses) there is a two and one-half page discussion of "headache" with brief mention of many specific causes (exogenous and endogenous toxins, skull disease, refractive error, sexual excesses [!]). The author states "In a majority of cases the headache occurs from neurasthesia, hysteria, and hemicrania (referring to the previous discussion of migraine.) ... Habitual or chronic headache is not rarely a chronic trouble that lasts for years, even for life."

Gowers (9) in 1898 discusses migraine in 20 pages, and then devotes another 6 pages to the "discussion of other headache". In this section he amplifies on the possible mechanism of pain, and devotes brief paragraphs to toxemia, gastric disturbances, "brain work and brain exhaustion" and neurasthesia. Another brief section discusses "head pressure and cephalic sensations." Neither are defined as causing a specific headache pattern.

It was undoubtedly the work of Harold Wolff's group in New York that had the most profound influence on the formulation of current concepts. In his monumental book (41), Wolff marshalled the evidence that induced "stressful" stimuli – painful injections to the scalp, pressure devices to the scalp – can produce secondarily muscle contraction which, he postulated, was in itself painful. Additional theory was that the muscle pain was derived from muscle ischemia secondary to long duration contraction. Wolff's formulation of the existence of "sustained contraction of muscle ... a source of pain and paresthesia of the head in tense, dissatisfied, apprehensive, anxious people" became generally accepted because of the detail of these experiments, and the link between "sustained contraction of muscle" and "tense ... people" was forged in medical literature without specific studies as to this relationship.

Also influential on subsequent thought was Sainsbury and Gibson's work (32), published in 1954, in which muscle tension in various muscles was recorded in 30 "anxious and tense" patients. It was reported that there were correlations between several symptoms (of which headache was one) and the degree of measured involuntary muscle tension; specifically onset of headache during recordings was "accompanied by significant increase in contraction of the frontalis muscle."

Diagnostic Problems

Recent work, to be discussed later, has raised problems as to the identity of this group of cases, and the etiology of the pain. The distinction from common migraine has proven difficult. Despite these uncertainties, it is apparent that the number of cases often diagnosed as suffering from "muscle contraction headache" is large. While most population surveys have concluded that migraine occurs in from 5 to 10% of those sampled, "severe headache" has been reported in the American population as occurring at some period in life in approximately 40-50% of those questioned (42). The prevalence of the problem in other societies has not often been studied but "migraine" strictly defined may have a fairly constant prevalence.

The original formulation of the concept of muscle contraction headaches must now be rethought for a variety of reasons. Current problems surrounding the subject may be summarized under eight questions.

QUESTIONS CONCERNING MUSCLE CONTRACTION HEADACHE:

1. Is there more tonic neck and scalp muscle contraction in patients so diagnosed than in controls?   -- in the migrainous?
2. Does muscle contraction in scalp or neck muscle increase parallel to pain?
3. During headache, is there more muscle contraction in patients so diagnosed than in the migrainous?
4. Do patients so diagnosed react to "stress" differently than controls?
5. What is the relation between psychological "tension" and muscle contraction headache?
6. What is the relation between muscle contraction headache and migraine?
7. Is muscle biofeedback effective?
8. Is muscle biofeedback specifically effective -- vs., e.g., relaxation exercises, other kinds of non-pharmacological treatment?

First to be considered is the question of whether patients so diagnosed do have excessive tension in neck or scalp muscles at rest. There have been several studies; the majority have not been able to confirm the fact that headache patient groups show on measurement more such neck or scalp muscle contraction than headache-free controls (36).

On balance furthermore the literature has not supported the concept that patients diagnosed as suffering from muscle contraction headache carry tonically more neck or scalp muscle contraction than the patients with other headache diagnoses (1,2,21,28,31).

If muscle contraction headache is a valid concept, increased tension in scalp and neck muscles should parallel severity of headache. Philips and Hunter carefully sift the evidence on this question and list seven studies that have not found such coincidence (29). Several articles have documented the heterogeneity of cases diagnosed "muscle contraction" and the fact that in a large percentage there is no correlation between level of neck or scalp EMG contraction and headache (24,26,36,38).

Several studies have addressed the hypothesis that the muscle contraction headache patients have an abnormal painful response to normal contraction, but there is no consistent evidence that "muscle contraction headache" patients react to stressful stimuli to a degree greater than controls, most studies being flawed by reason of (a) the use of a "stressful" stimulus that was not truly stressful to the patient, and (b) inadequate period of time for observation. Clearly further study is required.

Even more interesting is the study of muscle contraction as it relates to the clinical diagnosis of migraine, several studies showing that muscle contraction occurs during headache to an equal, sometimes greater, degree in patients clinically diagnosed as migraine than in those diagnosed as "muscle contraction" (1,2,31). Tender neck muscles are also common in migrainous patients, and injection of tender points (with local anesthetic or saline) has led to freedom from symptoms (37).

Much evidence then points to the conclusion that the concept of a symptomatic entity — muscle contraction headache — distinct from common migraine and due to muscle tension, needs to be dismantled and the facts reassembled. This conclusion accords with the intuition of many clinicians whose experience is that the diagnosis of migraine is usually easy, but that of "muscle contraction" headache difficult. The use of the category of "mixed" headache probably avoids this issue.

There are specific case reports in which striking rises in levels of muscle tension occur stimultaneously with occurrence of headache, but the concept of muscle contraction headache has been over-used and applied to large numbers of patients in whom it is not operative; it is possible that in small numbers of as yet poorly defined cases, muscle contraction may be etiologic or, in some patients, may be a "trigger" factor — perhaps related chiefly to the duration of such contraction. Finally, it is the feeling of some that more work devoted to the study of muscle contraction in the resting state, or as correlated with headache, is unnecessary. It is postulated that some, possibly few, headache-prone individuals are hyper-reactors to particular stressful stimuli and that attempts to identify these individuals would be fruitful. Such individuals might be those particularly benefiting by "desensitization" or various muscle relaxation training techniques, including biofeedback.

It seems unwise to base the diagnosis of muscle contraction headache on (a) lack of typical migrainous features and, (b) occipital, unusual or generalized head pain, since neither of these reliably identify a case group. Weinfeld of the U. S. National Institutes of Health analyzed, using a statistical factor analysis, a large group of headache patients. While classical and common migraine factors could be identified easily, muscle contraction or tension headache could not (39).

Another study with factor analysis found similar results (43). The artificiality of dividing patient groups into "muscle contraction" and "common migraine" is further attested to by the strikingly variable life course of headache-prone individuals. The usual history is that patients will have (a) single headache episodes with some of the characteristics ascribed to each diagnosis, and (b) at one time have typical migraine attacks, another time headache of "mixed type", and yet a third headache with most of the features of muscle contraction. In a Japanese study of patients attending various headache clinics, the percentage diagnosed as migraine varied from 5% to 34%, and those diagnosed as "tension" from 23% to 75% (12).

Psychological Characteristics

Psychological variables are usually used in the definition of muscle contraction headaches but there have been few systematic studies, although there is an immense literature on this subject, much of it highly controversial. Selby and Lance (33) estimated one-third of their patients "tense and anxious"; Dalsgard-Nielsen reported one-third of his headache patients with moderate, one-third with extreme "personality traits of sensitivity and perfectionism". Harrison (10) reviewed several studies; four reported fairly high degrees of neuroticism; but there have been negative studies in which no more neuroticism has been found in patients than controls (23). This last study showed, however, that these patients have certain personality traits, e.g., "elevated achievement, motivation, rigidity, fear of failure". On the MMPI test, "muscle contraction" patients have tended to show elevated score on hypochondriasis and hysteria (35). Depression has been found to be characteristic of the headache-prone population, but whether it is tied specifically to features of migraine or to severe headache in general is not well defined. While reports of head pain do not run parallel to the degree of muscle contraction in patients diagnosed as having muscle contraction headache, such pain is related to certain personality measures, specifically to "hypochondriasis" and conversion hysteria as measured on the MMPI scale (10).

With one exception there is little practical value in formal psychological testing in this group of patients. As noted above, most systematic studies have found more abnormalities in series of headache-prone patients than in controls, but such abnormalities have not distinguished clinically diagnosed migraine from muscle contraction headache. The exception, as noted above, is the importance of the detection of depression which is frequently associated with headache. The use of a simple questionnaire testing for depression (e.g., Zung) is helpful, not for a headache differential diagnosis but for detection of depression needing treatment. In a large unselected population studied with a headache questionnaire and two brief psychological tests, high scores on the Zung depression test were association with a history of "severe or disabling" headache to a statistically significant degree at all ages (44). A recent study of patients subjected to clinically diagnosed depressive disorder documents the circumstances of occurrence of headache with depressive episodes (8).

Diagnostic Tests

It is often difficult to judge when such patients need other tests to rule out organic disease. In general, the clues to organic disease causing headache are: (a) the appearance in an adult of a severe long-lasting headache with no previous history or precipitating cause; (b) severe headache persisting through all working hours. All patients of course must have a complete physical and neurological examination. Any abnormalities on the neurological examination, e.g., reflex asymmetry, mandate a search for intracranial disease.

Because of the absence of any reliable test for these headache syndromes, the clinician frequently orders diagnostic tests to reveal organic disease but this is rarely found. This caveat applies particularly to the use of computerized tomographic scanning of the head in patients diagnosed as having muscle contraction headache. Probably the only generalizations that can be made are (a) there should not be a "reflex" order of this procedure on each patient complaining of headache; and (b) as noted above, "different" headaches, and particularly those not responding to treatment, mandate the test. The clinician, of course, must accept, and instruct the patient to accept, the possibility of error.

A variety of systemic diseases - immunologic, vascular, infectious - may manifest themselves by headache; all patients with this complaint of any severity should have screening laboratory tests of blood count and the more routine blood chemistry studies.

Pain in the neck and back of the head is thought of as characteristic of muscle contraction headache. Similar pain can occur with cervical spine disease, particularly the common osteoarthritis. Pain elicited by movement gives a clue to this condition; when suspected, x-rays of the cervical spine are indicated and, occasionally, computerized tomography of that area.

Treatment

Treatment of episodic headache, whether the clinical diagnosis is migraine or muscle contraction headache, should begin with explanation to the patient that the physical and neurological examinations are normal. Many patients have the unexpressed apprehension that their head pain is the symptom of brain tumor or other dangerous brain disease. The extreme unlikelihood of this possibility should be stressed.

It is useful to give the patient a brief explanation of the state of knowledge in the field. Such explanation should include presentation of some of the medical controversies in the field – what is known and not known about the causes of pain. It is also helpful to tell patients that, in all pain problems, there is a mixture of "physical" and psychological elements. The explanation can then proceed to a discussion of the unpredictability of treatment results. The array of possible treatments – pharmacological and non-pharmacological – can be summarized with the statement that the tendency to headache is rarely "cured", but that the overall outlook for symptomatic help is good. Whatever the treatment, the physician should express interest in follow-up. Such an explanation diminishes the patient's passivity in treatment and enlists his/her cooperation. Finally, explanation of the difference between treatment of the attacks, and continuing prophylactic treatment should be given.

Simple analgesics, aspirin and acetaminophen are the pharmacological foundation of treatment for this type of headache. Patients should be told that (a) more than two aspirin tablets every four hours usually does not give additional analgesic effect; (b) aspirin can have a gastric irritant effect; and (c) continual use of very large amounts of acetaminophen can damage the kidneys. The use of more potent analgesics, e.g., opiates, especially by injection, is contraindicated, as the danger of habituation outweighs the value of any temporary effect.

Mild sedatives and tranquilizers potentiate analgesic effect, and small doses of acetaminophen or aspirin combined with a small amount of barbiturate are effective in the relief of a single headache attack. Many such medications also contain caffeine. Benzodiazepines can also be used for this purpose at the time of a severe headache.

The continued use of such medications on a regular daily basis is unwise. Large numbers of patients tend to increase the dosage taken and become dependent (3). The large amounts of caffeine ingested when these drugs are used with frequency can also lead to chronic headache and other symptoms.

Simple retreat to a quiet dark place with muscle relaxation should always be advised for the single attack.

For prophylaxis of recurrent attacks, amitriptyline has been reported successful in at least three studies. The original report of benefit of amitriptyline in patients with chronic tension headaches was by Lance in 1964 (20). Subsequently Diamond and Baltes (7) also reported, in a double-blind placebo-controlled study, the definite prophylactic effectiveness of the low dose of 10 mg in 90 patients "with anxiety or depression" who complained of headache. Pluvinage (30) has also reported good results with the drug in 53 out of 74 cases of tension headache, using varying dosage. Recently the effectiveness of another anti-depressant, femoxetine, which has a specific effect on the re-uptake of 5-hydroxytryptamine, has been reported effective in preventing headache in 16 patients diagnosed as tension headache in a double-blind placebo-controlled study (34). In view of the difficulty differentiating common migraine from muscle contraction headache episodes, propranolol in doses of 80-160 mg may also be tried, especially since several studies have reported its effectiveness in preventing anxiety attacks (17,18).

A variety of non-pharmacological treatments have been reported successful in training patients to avoid attacks. The early reports were of training in muscle relaxation. Instruction to these patients as to the importance of devoting regular periods of time to simple relaxation is undoubtedly important.

In the past twenty years there has been great interest in the efficacy of biofeedback – techniques in which the amount of muscle contraction, as recorded by surface electrodes, is displayed to the patient. The patient can then see his/her success or failure in achieving such relaxation. In the study of patients with headache, at times the frontalis muscle, and at others the neck muscles, have been studied. A large body of literature has accumulated concerning this popular treatment in recent years, and while certain facts about it seem to have become established, others are controversial.

The first fact is that contraction at rest in the muscles studied can indeed be recorded and that patients can learn to relax these muscles. The weight of evidence is in favor of the statement that patients using EMG biofeedback treatment suffer fewer headaches and headaches of lesser intensity and duration than do non-treatment controls (13), but there have been two negative reports (5,14).

The critical questions in evaluating this treatment have always been whether (a) the specific achievement of muscle relaxation is the cause of improvement, as opposed to a subjective state ("relaxation") independent of muscle contraction; and (b) do patients using the biofeedback visualization do better than those without this addition to the effect of "training"?

As to the first problem, it has been repeatedly demonstrated, as discussed previously, that a considerable percentage of patients diagnosed as muscle contraction headache do not have, both in headache and non-headache periods, greater amounts of neck or scalp muscle contraction than other groups. It is difficult to postulate muscle relaxation as the therapeutic element in this group.

Concerning the question as to whether patients learning "relaxation" do better with visualization of muscle contraction, at least three studies came to the conclusion that muscle biofeedback is not superior to relaxation training (6,11,40). Muscle relaxation treatment has been "successful" with no change in headache sensation (40).

These negative studies have in turn been criticized because (a) many of them used the frontalis muscle as the element studied, whereas the neck muscles are those most closely associated with headache (15); and (b) training courses of intensive nature have been successful while those of more prolonged duration have not. In some cases progressive relaxation treatment was successful whereas biofeedback was not.

Biofeedback training was initially applied to blood flow – learning to raise finger temperature – a maneuver thought to diminish cerebral blood flow and therefore to be beneficial in migraine. Since the distinction between migraine and muscle contraction headache has been blurred, its efficacy in muscle contraction headache is worthy of comment. It has been established that certain individuals can raise finger temperature, but early studies were uncontrolled and in a careful review of the subject Holmes and Burish (13) concluded that in none of the four recent controlled studies was there evidence of a specific therapeutic effect on migraine of learning elevation of finger temperature. In reports of benefit from elevating finger temperature, patients diagnosed as migraine and those diagnosed as muscle contraction fared equally.

In a study by Philips and Hunter (27) of a group of patients who had been diagnosed as "chronic tension headaches" but who had been found to lack any abnormality in scalp or neck muscle tension, patients were given instruction in general relaxation, combined in one group with visual imagery – but with no biofeedback. One-quarter became symptom free, and half the cases improved by 66%. The authors comment that biofeedback itself may be counter productive in reducing headaches, in contrast to general relaxation techniques.

There have been very few studies comparing pharmacological to non-pharmacological treatments in these patients, but one compared biofeedback to "the most suitable alternative therapy" which was either "physical therapy or drugs (analgesics, sedatives, anti-depressants or muscle relaxants) alone or in combination." Results showed significant improvement in headache intensity, severity and drug intake in the feedback group only (4). One more placebo-controlled study compared the use of diazepam and frontal EMG biofeedback in tension headache (25). Both were found to be effective, although with different timings. Diazepam was more effective during treatment, but treatment effects were briefer than with biofeedback. This study also found a lack of correlation between frontalis muscle tension and the degree of headache. In another study comparing the effectiveness of biofeedback in patients who were or were not receiving concomitant pharmacotherapy, it was found that both amitriptyline and propranolol made the response to biofeedback training much more variable (16).

There has been much interest in recent years in acupuncture as a treatment for chronic pain. Although it is generally acknowledged that pain relief occurs, there remains debate as to whether results from placement of the needles in the traditional points is superior to that of placement in other arbitrarily chosen points, i.e., a suitable placebo control. Most of the studies have been done on patients with back and other skeletal pain. An Australian study commented that to the date of publication (January, 1983) there had been six reported trials using a controlled double-blind protocol, of which four had found acupuncture not superior to placebo, and the Australian study added a further one to that number. Acupuncture specifically for headache has rarely been studied systematically, although one report on migraine was positive (19).

Acknowledgements:

This project was partially supported by funds from the National Migraine Foundation, Chicago, Illinois, and Marion Laboratories of Kansas City, Missouri. Gratitude is expressed to Patricia Melching and Althea Ballenger for assistance in the typing of this manuscript.

REFERENCES

1. Anderson, C., and Franks, R. D. (1981): Headache, 21:63.
2. Bakal, D. A., and Kaganov, J. A. (1977): Headache, 17:308.
3. Brill, H. (1972): JAMA, 220:1018.
4. Bruhn, P., Olesen, J., and Melgaard, B. (1979): Ann. Neurol., 6:34.
5. Chesney, M. A., and Shelton, J. L. (1976): J. Behav. Ther. Exp. Psychiat., 7:221.
6. Cox, D. J., Freundlich, A., and Meyer, R. G. (1975): J. Consult. Clin. Psychol., 43:892.
7. Diamond, S., and Baltes, B. J.: Headache, 110-116.
8. Garvey, M. J., Schaffer, C. B., and Tuason, V. B. (1983): Brit. J. Psychiat., 143:544.
9. Gowers, W. R. (1898): Diseases of the Nervous System, Volume 2. B. Blakiston, Son & Co., Philadelphia.
10. Harrison, R. H. (1975): Headache, 177-184.
11. Haynes, S. N., Griffin, P., Mooney, D., and Parise, M. (1975): Behav. Ther., 6:672.
12. Hirayama, K., and Ito, N. (1982): In: Advances in Migraine Research and Therapy, edited by F. C. Rose, pp. 13-23. Raven Press, New York.
13. Holmes, D. S., and Burish, T. G.: (1983): J. Psychosomat. Res., 27:515.
14. Holroyd, K. A., Andrasik, F., and Westbrook, T. (1977): Cognitive Ther. Res., 1:121.
15. Hudzinski, L. G. (1983): Headache, 23:86.
16. Jay, G. W., Renelli, D., and Mead, T. (1984): Headache, 24:59.
17. Kathol, R., Noyes, R., Jr., Slymen, D. J., Crowe, R. R., Clancy, J., and Kerber, R. E. (1980): Arch. Gen. Psychiat., 37:1361.
18. Kellner, R., Collins, A. C., Shulman, R. S., and Pathak, D. (1974): J. Clin. Pharmacol., 5:301.
19. Kim, K. C., and Yount, R. A. (1974): Amer. J. Chinese Med., 2:407.
20. Lance, J. W., Sydney, M. D., and Curran, D. A. (1964): Lancet; June 6.
21. Martin, P. R., and Mathews, A. M. (1978): J. Psychosom. Res., 22:389.
22. Oppenheim, H. (1900): Diseases of the Nervous System, translated by Edward E. Mayer. J. B. Lippincott Company, Philadelphia and London.
23. Passchier, J., van der Helm-Hylkema, H., and Oriebeke, J. F. (1984): Headache, 24:140.
24. Passchier, M. D., van der Helm-Hylkema, H., and Oriebeke, J. F. (1984): Headache, 24:131.
25. Paiva, T., Nunes, J. S., Moreira, A., Santos, J., Teixeira, J., and Barbosa, A. (1982): Headache, 22:216.
26. Philips, C., and Hunter, M. (1981): Behav. Res. Ther., 19:485.

27. Philips, C., and Hunter, M. (1981): Behav. Res. Ther., 19:499.
28. Philips, H. C., and Hunter, M. S. (1982): Headache, 22:173.
29. Pikoff, H. (1984): Headache, 24:186.
30. Pluvinage, R. (1978): Sem. Hop. Paris., 54(21-24):713-716. 8-15 Sep. 1978.
31. Pozniak-Patewicz, E. (1976): Headache, 15:261.
32. Sainsbury, P., and Gibson, J. G. (1954): J. Neurol. Neurosurg. Psychiat., 17:216.
33. Selby, G., and Lance, J. W. (1960): J. Neurol. Neurosurg. Psychiat., 23:23.
34. Sjaastad, O. (1983): Cephalagia, 3:53.
35. Sternbach, R. A., Dalessio, D. J., Kunzel, M., and Bowman, G. E. (1980): Headache, 20:311.
36. Sutton, E. R., and Belar, C. D. (1981): Headache, 21:63.
37. Tfelt-Hansen, P., Lous, I., and Olesen, J. (1981): Headache, 21:49.
38. Turkat, I. E. (1980): Degree dissertation, University of Georgia, Athens Georgia. University Microfilms (publication No. 80-29161), Ann Arbor, Michigan.
39. Weinfeld, F. D., and Richter, R. (1984): Paper delivered at the annual meeting of the American Association for the Study of Headache, San Francisco, California, June 23, 1984.
40. Wieselberg Bell, N., Abramowitz, S. I., Folkins, C. H., Spensley, J., and Hutchinson, G. L. (1983): Headache, 23:162.
41. Wolff, H. G. (1963): Headache and Other Head Pain, 2nd Edition. Oxford University Press, New York.
42. Ziegler, D. K., Hassanein, R. S., and Couch, J. R. (1977): Neurology, 27:265.
43. Ziegler, D. K., Hassanein, R. S., and Couch, J. R. (1982): Cephalagia, 2:125.
44. Ziegler, D. K., Rhoades, R. J., and Hassanein, R. S. (1966): Headache, 6:123.

The Management of Headache, edited
by F. Clifford Rose. Raven Press,
New York © 1988.

HEADACHE IN THE EMERGENCY DEPARTMENT

John Edmeads, MD

Professor of Neurology, Sunnybrook Medical Center,
University of Toronto, Ontario M4N 3M5, Canada

People with headaches come to the Emergency Department for
one of two reasons. Either the headache is the most recent in a
seemingly endless series of similar headaches, so that the
patient presents because of frustration, exhaustion or despair
(the "last straw" syndrome); or the headache is sufficiently
different or sufficiently severe to alarm the patient (the
"first or the worst" syndrome).

The two syndromes differ in presentation, significance, and
management.

The "Last Straw" Syndrome

These patients have a long history of chronic recurring
headaches -- migraine, tension ("muscle contraction"), or a
mixture of the two. Typically the headaches have not been well
controlled; they have been increasing in frequency, duration
and/or severity; and the patient is having increasing problems
with medication, with their own reactions to their headaches,
and with those "significant others" with whom they and their
headaches interact. In short, these patients present largely
because of emotional decompensation.

Familiar scenarios are: (a) the patient who has had a
headache for hours or days, has consumed a large quantity of
analgesics, has run out of medication, and who now presents to
the Emergency Department (often in the evening or night-time
hours) with a demand for instant relief, preferably from "a
needle"; and (b) the patient who has made things so difficult
for family or friends that he/she is deposited in the Emergency
Department with poorly concealed exasperation and the plea
"please fix the headaches!".

Only a small minority of patients with chronic recurrent
headaches frequent Emergency Departments. Those who do, tend to
share certain characteristics.

In terms of emotional state: (a) anxiety and depression
are almost invariable accompaniments of the headache, and often
there is doubt in the physician's mind as to which is cause, and

139

which effect; (b) hypochondriasis (a compulsive preoccupation with, and an ordering of the universe in terms of, symptoms) is frequent; (c) manipulative behavior (a tendency to use symptoms to control the environment) is occasionally evident.

Medication problems are the rule, and include: (a) emotional or physical dependence upon analgesics and/or sedatives, with consequent "medication-seeking behavior"; (b) tolerance to analgesics, so that the patient consumes larger and larger amounts in a vain effort to restore a dwindling therapeutic effect; (c) rebound cycles involving one or more of codeine, barbiturate, ergotamine or caffeine; as the time from the last dose increases, blood levels of these substances fall, provoking withdrawal symptoms which may include headache, leading to consumption of more medication, and locking the patient within a cycle.

The total picture presented by these patients with the "last straw" syndrome is daunting. It is not realistic to expect the emergency physician to provide a final solution to such a longstanding and complex problem, particularly in the setting of a busy, sometimes hectic Emergency Department. Reasonable objectives are: (a) to provide a brief haven for the patient from the situation that may have provoked or perpetuated that attack of headache; (b) to reduce the pain, vomiting, anxiety and other symptoms produced by the attack; and (c) to arrange referral for definitive longterm treatment of the patient and his/her headaches.

Pain reduction can be a challenging problem. Clearly, ergotamine is contraindicated in this situation. It is far too late for it to be helpful, and used at this stage it can do nothing but increase nausea and vomiting. There is a temptation to use narcotics, but often these are not very effective. Almost always the patient has been taking codeine (a weak narcotic) at home, or perhaps somewhat stronger narcotics such as pentazocine or oral meperidine, and their failure is attested by the patient's presence in the Emergency Department. There are a number of possible reasons for this not infrequent inefficacy of narcotics. A sophisticated (and unproven) explanation is presented below (see Status Migrainosus). A more down-to-earth formulation is that in these "last straw" patients the pain is at least as much emotional as it is physical. Certainly, powerful tranquilizing agents such as chlorpromazine or methotrimeprazine, in a dose of 25-50 mg intramuscularly, usually work much better than narcotics to reduce pain, nausea, vomiting and agitation. They settle the patient down smoothly and -- a not unimportant consideration -- their use, rather than that of a narcotic, settles any nagging doubts the physician may have that he could be giving narcotics to an addict who is simulating migraine in order to obtain morphine or meperidine.

Most patients with the "last straw" syndrome can be given adequate relief in the course of a relatively brief (a few hours) stay in the Emergency Department, and then can be returned home in the care of family and friends, with instructions on how and where to secure definitive longterm treatment for their headache problem.

There is one group of patients within the "last straw" syndrome who, while they resemble in some respects all other patients in that rubric (e.g., long history of migraine headaches, deteriorating control of symptoms, problems with medication, etc.), differ in one significant respect -- they are acutely physically ill. These are the patients in "status migrainosus". There is no universally accepted definition of status migrainosus, but the essential elements (3) appear to be: (a) a true migraine (as opposed to "muscle contraction") headache; (b) of long duration (usually 72 hours or more); (c) refractory to self-administered medications (analgesics, etc.); and (d) producing sufficient true disability or debilitation that presentation to hospital is genuinely indicated.

Patients in status migrainosus are truly miserable. Not only are they in severe pain in addition to emotional distress, but nausea and vomiting may produce dehydration and electrolyte imbalance. In contrast to most patients with the "last straw" syndrome, patients in status migrainosus often require hospitalization.

If possible, these patients should be put to rest in a quiet, semi-darkened environment. Dehydration and electrolyte imbalance from vomiting or from profuse sweating require intravenous fluid therapy. Many clinicians insert an intravenous line in all status migrainosus patients; it serves as a route for administration of some medications, and it is a wise precaution when using agents that may be complicated by hypotension.

As noted previously, pain relief poses special problems. Some clinicians feel that in many patients with migraine, parenteral opioids such as meperidine or morphine are not helpful; either the injection does not ease the pain at all, serving only to increase nausea and vomiting, or it produces only transient benefit. It has been speculated that because opiate analgesia may be dependent upon the integrity of a serotoninergic projection of the nucleus raphe magnus (1), and because migraine may be a state characterized by depletion of central nervous system serotonin, then opiates are incapable of producing effective analgesia for attacks of migraine. Opposed to this speculation is the observation that at least some patients do obtain adequate relief from the pain of migraine with parenteral narcotics.

Reservations about the efficacy of narcotics have produced a trend towards the use of powerful phenothiazines for the treatment of status migrainosus and, properly administered, these seem to work as well as or better than opiates for many patients. Chlorpromazine 25-50 mg (for an average-sized otherwise healthy adult) injected deeply intramuscularly, can settle anxiety, nausea, vomiting and pain quickly and effectively. In some Emergency Departments it is customary to give 12.5-25 mg chlorpromazine intravenously (slowly, through an injection into the intravenous tubing of a normal saline drip); this can allay pain, fear and vomiting quite dramatically but has the disadvantage of producing hypotension. However, these patients are supine in any event because of their symptoms, so hypotension seldom is a problem. Clearly it is prudent to keep all patients who have received parenteral phenothiazines supine for four hours, and to follow their blood pressure half-hourly throughout that interval. Methotrimeprazine may be more effective than chlorpromazine because of its reputed intrinsic analgesic properties; dosage ranges from 12.5-50 mg intramuscularly; again, hypotension may occur.

Some clinicians use parenteral corticosteroids (2,4), either alone or in combination with other medications, to terminate status migrainosus. This treatment is empirical, and probably derives from the traditional role of corticosteroids as the pharmacological last rites for neurological disease. There is no compelling rationale for their use, though some claim that they act by reducing inflammation in blood vessels and by sensitizing blood vessels to the vasoconstrictive effects of circulating catecholamines. Despite the lack of rationale, many clinicians are convinced that they are effective. Some regimens used are: (a) hydrocortisome sodium succinate 100-250 mg by slow injection (over about ten minutes) into the intravenous tubing of a drip of normal saline, or (b) dexamethasone sodium phosphate 12-20 mg intramuscularly or intravenously. A repeat parenteral dose, or its oral equivalent, may be necessary in 8-12 hours, but corticosteroid treatment beyond 24 hours is a step that requires very careful consideration. In general, if corticosteroids have not terminated status migrainosus in 24 hours, they are unlikely to do so later.

Rest, hydration, phenothiazines and corticosteroids, together with the intangible but essential elements of support and reassurance, bring the majority of patients through an attack of status migrainosus quickly.

Most experienced clinicians avoid ergotamine and dihydroergotamine (DHE) in treating status migrainosus; almost always, it is far too late for these. There is controversy about the use of "cocktails" of barbiturates and phenothiazines to induce sleep and thus terminate headache. What these cocktails may induce is not sleep, but general anesthesia, and the clinician must balance the risks of this against those of less drastic but equally effective measures.

The "First or the Worst" Syndrome

These patients may or may not have a history of recurrent headaches. Among those who do not are some who present with what is clearly a first attack of either common or classic migraine. It is usual to encounter people with a first attack of common migraine in the Emergency Department; more often they cope with that headache themselves at home; using over-the-counter analgesics, and then present to their family doctors. Possibly the ubiquity of commercials for headache medication conditions our populace to the apparent inevitability of headaches, so that they are not particularly alarmed when they experience one, providing it is not too severe.

But a first attack of classic migraine, with its conspicuous neurological accompaniments, is much more likely to alarm the patient and lead to presentation to the Emergency Department. Almost always, these first attacks of classic migraine cause no diagnostic difficulty, and respond well to explanation, reassurance, rest, analgesic and antiemetic treatment.

In contrast, a first attack of a rare variety of migraine, such as cheiro-oral migraine, hemiplegic migraine, basilar migraine or ophthalmoplegic migraine, inevitabily produces severe problems in diagnosis and usually calls for specialized neurological investigation. The prominent neurological signs or symptoms that accompany these migraine variants ensure that the emergency physician will not dismiss these patients lightly. Cheiro-oral migraine, with its spreading hand-and-face paresthesias, may mimic focal sensory seizures or transient cerebral ischemia. Hemiplegic and basilar migraine, with their focal neurological deficits and ensuing headaches, may suggest the diagnoses of cerebral embolism, brain tumor, arteriovenous malformation, or subdural hematoma. The headache and unilateral oculomotor palsy of ophthalmoplegic migraine raises the spectre of a leaking aneurysm or of transtentorial hippocampal herniation or, less ominously, diabetic ophthalmoplegia. Though frightening and complex, these syndromes present such a florid picture and occasion such vigorous investigation that neither they nor any of the diseases they mimic are likely to remain undiagnosed for long.

Much more difficult to diagnose is the patient, with or without a history of prior headaches, who presents with "the worst headache ever". True, those patients who are brought into the Emergency Department with collapse, obtunded consciousness, board-like nuchal rigidity, subhyaloid hemorrhages, and a neurological deficit, are diagnostic child's play. However, a full house is as rare in medicine as it is in poker; and for every patient in the Emergency Department with a textbook picture of subarachnoid hemorrhage, there are a dozen who present only with the sudden onset of a very severe headache, with minimal or no stiffness of the neck, and with no abnormal neurological signs. Which of these patients have "just a severe migraine" and which have a leaking berry aneurysm -- or meningitis? How much investigation is it reasonable to do in order to detect or rule out these ominous possibilities?

The dimensions of the problem are suggested by the following: Every year in North America 28,000 people suffer rupture of an intracranial aneurysm. Of these, 7,000 have warning signals ignored, are initially misdiagnosed, and/or are referred too late for surgery to help (6). In the experience of one major U.S. medical center (7), if every patient who presented with acute severe headache and no other findings received a CT scan to search for subarachnoid hemorrhage, the cost (at 1977 prices) of identifying one patient with subarachnoid hemorrhage would be $32,895. If CT scanning were reserved for those with acute severe headache and abnormal neurological signs, then the cost of identifying one case of subarachnoid hemorrhage would fall to $1,050., but this is the group in which diagnosis is least difficult. CT scans may fail to detect up to 10% of all cases of subarachnoid hemorrhage (8); and CT scans may be normal in early uncomplicated meningitis (5).

To the question of how to distinguish effectively and economically between the benign headache of severe migraine and the malignant headache of subarachnoid hemorrhage or of meningitis, there is no perfect answer. A workable solution involves: (a) identifying within the large group of "emergency headache patients" those individuals more likely to be harboring serious disease; and (b) investigating those individuals with procedures most likely to identify and least likely to miss serious disease.

Identification of these individuals requires a very high order of history-taking and physical examination skills. Those points in history most sensitive in terms of suggesting the presence of a lesion are: (a) Relationship of onset to exertion. While it is true that there are such things as "effort-induced migraine" and "coital cephalalgia", and while it is true that aneurysms may rupture during sleep, it is also true that all these occurrences are unusual. Onset of headache during exertion suggests subarachnoid hemorrhage. (b) Altered awareness. It is said that during a severe migraine headache, sufferers may faint or become confused, and it is beyond dispute that some people may remain alert despite clear-cut subarachnoid hemorrhage or meningitis, but in general, confusion and obtundation are much more typical of subarachnoid hemorrhage or meningitis than of migraine. (c) Posterior radiation of pain. Migraine may be associated with nucho-occipital pain which has been ascribed to muscle contraction, but pain between the shoulder blades, or lower, is very suggestive of subarachnoid blood or pus tracking along the spinal theca. (d) Prior or coexistent infectious disease. A respiratory or gastrointestinal infection may trigger an attack of migraine, but much more significant is the possibility that an infection elsewhere in the body may have led to meningitis. Obfuscating diagnosis at this point is the consideration of "toxic vascular headache". Some people with febrile infectious illnesses may have very severe diffuse headaches of sudden onset, and may even exhibit some slight limitation of passive forward flexion of the neck. Lumbar puncture (mandatory in this setting) yields perfectly normal cerebrospinal fluid, and the headache then fades as fever and the systemic infection settle. The important principle is that fever is not part of migraine, and the presence of fever or infection demands further investigation to search for meningitis. (Fever may occur in subarachnoid hemorrhage, but usually not until the second or third day following the hemorrhage.) (e) Age of the patient. While the first attack of migraine can occur as late as age 50, and while an aneurysm may rupture in the teens or twenties, these are unusual events. Most first attacks of migraine occur before the age of 30, and most aneurysms rupture after the age of 30. Abrupt onset of severe headache in a 40 year old with no previous history of headache should suggest an ominous cause.

Physical examination often is said to be normal in these individuals with their "worst headache ever" but sometimes careful re-examination will yield abnormal signs which will raise the level of suspicion of ominous disease. (a) Stiff neck. In eliciting this sign, technique is everything. It is very common for experienced clinicians to detect slight degrees of nuchal rigidity that have been missed by house officers. Gentleness is essential. Have the patient as relaxed as possible. With hand under occiput, flex the neck foward slowly and evenly, observing the patient's face for the first sign of additional discomfort, observing the legs for the involuntary flexion that relieves the stretch on inflamed spinal meninges, and staying alert for the slight "catch" in the forward traverse of the neck that denotes meningeal irritation. Repeat the test at intervals, for the onset of signs of meningeal irritation may be delayed. (Meningeal irritation may be absent in the very young, the very old, and the very sick, but the presence of serious disease is not usually in doubt in these situations.) (b) General appearance of the patient. Patients with an attack of migraine may look quite ill, and patients with a small subarachnoid hemorrhage or early meningitis may seem deceptively well. It is a matter of nice judgment to determine whether a patient is "sicker than he should be for migraine", and often this judgment is made by gut feeling rather than by conscious ratiocination. Nevertheless, an experienced clinician (i.e., one who has made lots of mistakes) can use this effectively as a pointer to the presence of serious disease. (c) Soft signs. Penalties of the age of neurotechnology are the atrophy of clinical skills and the forgetting that the single best neurological investigation is a repeat history and examination. (Contrary to the dictum of a prominent Texas surgeon, "a C.A.T. scan is worth a roomful of neurologists" only some of the time.) The initial examinaiton may not truly have been normal, and a repeat examination done with care may elicit subtle abnormalities such as slight pupillary inequality, slight drift of an outstretched limb, slight asymmetry of plantar responses, or slight confusion. The finding of any abnormality, however subtle, places the patient into a "greater risk" group for whom investigation is mandatory.

Using all these criteria the clinician can place his "worst headache ever" patients into one of two categories.

Young people who may have had a previous history of headaches, or who have a family history of headaches; who have come to the Emergency Department with severe headache but are beginning to settle down; who have no suspicious factors in history (see above); who are, and have been, perfectly alert and oriented; who on repeated examinations have no neurological abnormalities, no fever, and no evidence of meningeal irritation -- these are in a low risk category. They may reasonably be observed without further investigation; be given treatment for an acute attack of migraine; and, if they improve, be sent home in custody of family or friends.

All other patients fall into a high risk category, and are managed as follows: (a) If there is papilledema, if there is impairment of consciousness or of orientation, or if there are localizing or lateralizing neurological signs, then a CT scan should be done immediately. If a CT scan is not available, then the patient should be transferred urgently to a facility where a CT scan can be obtained. Isotope scans and angiograms are usually second best to a CT scan for identifying or ruling out, in this situation, intracerebral or extracerebral hematoma, brain abscess, other space-taking lesions, and hydrocephalus. If any of these lesions are found, neurosurgical assistance should be sought. Note that there are limitations of a CT scan. A normal CT scan does not rule out a small subarachnoid hemorrhage and should not be used for this purpose. Nor does a normal CT scan exclude early uncomplicated meningitis. Only lumbar puncture will do these. (b) If the CT scan done in the above circumstances is normal, or if the patient has none of the features that would call for a CT scan to be done, lumbar puncture should be performed. The purposes of the lumbar puncture are to establish the presence or absence of blood or inflammatory cells in the cerebrospinal fluid (CSF); to differentiate between subarachnoid hemorrhage and meningitis in a patient with a stiff neck and no other neurological signs; and to determine the etiologic agent when meningitis is present.

Lumbar puncture is a readily available and inexpensive investigation. It is also invasive, uncomfortable, and capable of causing enormous diagnostic confusion when inexpertly done, and it is therefore essential that it not be botched. It should be done by the most experienced person available, to minimize the occurrence of a "bloody tap". The CSF pressure should always be measured, since this may be the first indication that intracranial pressure is raised (an embarrassing but not dangerous situation, provided that the lumbar puncture has been done on patients selected as above). Even if crystal clear, the CSF should immediately be examined under the microscope for cells, preferably by the clinician (who is likely to have more experience in identifying cells in CSF than a junior laboratory technician). If the CSF is bloody, it should be collected in three tubes, and cells should be counted in the first and third tubes. A decrease in erythrocyte count from first to third tubes suggests an artefactual bloody tap; an increase suggests genuine subarachnoid hemorrhage. The bloody CSF should be centrifuged, and the supernatant examined for xanthochromia. A common error is to send the CSF to the laboratory to be centrifuged, rather than doing this on the spot in the Emergency Department. A delay in getting the CSF to the laboratory, and the jostling of the specimen in transit, may lyse erythrocytes that have been put there by the lumbar puncture needle, producing xanthochromia that cannot be distinguished from that caused by lysis of erythrocytes from a subarachnoid hemorrhage, and hopelessly confusing the diagnosis.

The clinician should not let the CSF out of his custody until he has satisfied himself in the Emergency Department that one of four circumstances exist: (a) There are no cells in the CSF, and therefore the patient is extremely unlikely to have either subarachnoid hemorrhage or meningitis, and should be managed as in an acute attack of migraine, or as a toxic vascular headache, and observed. (b) There are leucocytes in the CSF, and therefore the patient has meningitis and will be investigated urgently along these lines. (c) There are erythrocytes in the CSF which, because of an increasing count from first to third tubes, and because of xanthochromia, signify subarachnoid hemorrhage and the need for an emergency neurosurgical consultation; or (d) There are erythrocytes in the CSF which, because of a decreasing count from the first to the third tubes, and in the absence of xanthochromia, indicate an artefactually bloody tap; the patient should be managed as an acute migraine or toxic vascular headache, and observed.

The CSF may then be surrendered to the laboratory for confirmation of the above findings, and for determination of appropriate values such as sugar, protein, culture and sensitivities, etc.

This algorithm, carefully applied, will identify those patients in the "first or the worst" headache situation who have serious disease, and will point the way to appropriate treatment.

Summary

At any time headache is a challenging exercise in diagnosis and treatment. In the Emergency Department the difficulty and challenge are magnified by the acuteness and the severity of the headache and by the need for rapid, appropriate and safe management of the patient. Adherence to a few rational principles help ensure a satisfactory outcome for patients with "emergency headaches".

REFERENCES

1. Basbaum, A. I., and Fields, H. L. (1978): Ann. Neurol., 4:451.
2. Carroll, J. D. (1971): Brit. Med. J., 2:756.
3. Couch, J. R., and Diamond, S. (1983): Headache, 23:94.
4. Edmeads, J. (1973): Headache, 13:91.
5. Enzmann, D. R. (1984): In: Computed Tomography, Ultrasound, and Nuclear Magnetic Resonance, p. 190.   Raven Press, New York.
6. Kassell, N. F., and Drake, C. G. (1982): Neurosurgery, 10:514.
7. Knaus, W. A., Wagner, D. P., and Davis, D. O. (1981): Amer. J. Roentgenology, 136:537.
8. Scotti, G., Ethier, R., Melanen, D., Terbugge, K., and Tchang, S. (1977): Radiology, 123:85.

The Management of Headache, edited
by F. Clifford Rose. Raven Press,
New York © 1988.

HEADACHES IN CHILDREN

Judith Hockaday, MD, FRCP

Consultant in Paediatric Neurology,
John Radcliffe Hospital, Oxford, England

Headache is important in children, first because it may be
symptomatic of serious intracranial disease, and second because
it is an extremely common complaint.

It is customary to consider the subject according to
whether headache is an acute new symptom, or one in a series of
recurring attacks. The main causes of headache in children are
shown below.

TABLE 1.   Some Important Causes of Headaches in Children.

Acute:

           Constitutional
           Cranial infection
           Trauma (N.A.I.)
           Hemorrhage

Recurrent:

           Intracranial tumor
           Hydrocephalus
           Pseudotumor cerebri
           Hypertension
           Ocular - ENT - Dental
           Post-traumatic
           Epilepsy
           Depression

"Unexplained":

           Migraine
           Tension headache
           Psychogenic
           Conversion symptoms

Prevalence

All studies of headache prevalence in childhood agree in
finding it high (Table 2). Bille (5) observed that 59% of 8993

school children had experienced headaches, although they were infrequent in all except 10%. Sillanpaa (88) reported that 28% of 2915 children aged 14 experienced headache at least once a month. Waters (105) found that 27% of girls aged 10-16 had consulted their doctors at some time because of headache.

TABLE 2.   Prevalence of Headache in School Children.

Authors:	Year:	Age:	Boys:		Girls:
Bille	1962	7-15	58%		59%
Waters*	1974	10-16	85%		93%
Deubner	1977	10-15	74%		82%
Sillanpaa	1983	7		37%	
		14		69%	
Collin et al.	1984	9-12		76%	

*14% had consulted their doctor because of headache.

Acute Headache in a Previously Healthy Child

Constitutional Upset

This is probably the commonest cause of headache in children, where it can accompany fever of any cause (17). Although it may be the only symptom complained of, it is usually part of a recognizable clinical picture, which is apparent on general examination.

Intracranial Infection

Although drowsiness, irritability, and photophobia can occur in any child with fever, and in the course of severe migraine, they also suggest intracranial infection: bacterial and viral meningitis, encephalitis, intracranial abscess. They are thus indications for special investigation especially in a child with headache. Headache is a common early (prodromal) symptom in herpex simplex encephalitis. Symptoms of raised intracranial pressure (vomiting or alteration of conscious level), or evidence of focal neurological involvement suggest intracranial abscess: failure to demonstrate any infection source does not rule this out; sometimes all that is found is sinusitis (50). In subacute and chronic meningitis, headache is more insidious. Tuberculous meningitis is reported still in children (72), and in young children the history of headache, lethargy and anorexia may exceed three weeks (28).

Trauma

In younger children with head injury, trauma may not be remembered, and this will be the case at any age when there is retrograde amnesia. Every child presenting with headache must therefore be carefully examined for bruising. Non-accidental injury should be considered if the circumstances are unclear.

Roberton et al. (80) found head and facial bruising much more often in children in whom non-accidental injury was likely than in other traumatized children of the same age.

Occasionally minor trauma will cause hemorrhage from an underlying vascular malformation and this should be considered when headache of acute onset is prolonged, or increases in severity or when associated symptoms of neck stiffness, drowsiness or vomiting appear. Sometimes relatively minor trauma causes disruption of cerebrospinal fluid (CSF) dynamics, and leads to symptoms of headache, drowsiness and vomiting for the first time in children who have a previously balanced hydrocephalus either in relation to a space occupying lesion, or with so-called arrested congenital hydrocephalus (38). Demonstration of a large head size will be an important guide to the latter possibility.

Head injury (sometimes without obvious fracture) is a known cause predisposing to pneumococcal meningitis in children (97), perhaps by spread of infection across disrupted meninges; this possibility should be considered in a child whose headaches start, or increase, a few days after head trauma.

Hemorrhage

Spontaneous intracranial hemorrhage is rare in childhood. The Carlisle Survey (9) did not identify any cases of subarachnoid hemorrhage (SAH) in a five year period in the 0-19 year age group, and in a review of the literature found only eight (0.5%) of 1624 patients with SAH who were under ten years old. In one childhood series (86), the causes of hemorrhage were rupture of saccular aneurysm (in 27), vascular malformation (in 16), or unknown (in 24). Typical presentation is with headache of increasing severity and unresponsiveness to analgesics, followed by deterioration of conscious level.

Recurrent Headaches

Probably the majority of recurrent headaches in childhood are "unexplained" (Table 1) or are caused by relatively minor pathological lesions such as sinusitis, or ocular problems. A few are the result of serious neurological or psychiatric disease. The distinction is often difficult and generally much more care has to be taken in children and clinical investigation should be done more often and sooner than in adults.

Cerebral Tumor

Although cerebral tumor is rare (average annual incidence 5.2 per 100,000 population age 0-9 years in the Carlisle study, reference #9), it (together with tumors of the spinal cord) is the second commonest cause, after leukemia, of childhood malignancy (78). At all ages except infancy, headache is the most important symptom of brain tumor, especially of those in the posterior fossa where 45% of childhood brain tumors arise (85). Honig and Charney (49) found 72 out of 105 children with brain tumor had associated headaches, <u>which preceded neurological and/or ocular signs in at least 83%</u>. The headaches were occipital in 28%, unilateral in 22%, and diffuse in 50%. Skull x-ray was normal in 46% at time of diagnosis. The headache of brain tumor results from local traction, and from the indirect distorting effects of the hydrocephalus which is generally present by the time of diagnosis: Honig and Charney (49) recorded vomiting in 78% of children with brain tumor headache, and papilledema was present in 63% at time of diagnosis. Geissinger and Bucy (33) observed papilledema at presentation in 88% of children with cerebellar astrocytoma.

There may be no specific features about the headache of brain tumor. The course can be intermittent with long remissions and the headache can be mild. Distinction from migraine or muscle tension headache is often not possible from the character of the headache alone. The circumstances in which it occurs are more helpful; they include any cause of altered intracranial pressure such as cough, sneezing, straining, exercise, recumbency and sleep. Thus morning headache or headache which actually wakes a child can be ominous. Honig and Charney (49) observed this feature in 67% of their series. However, in a review of the characteristics of brain tumor headaches (all ages), Rushton and Rooke (84) found this feature in only 25% of cases overall.

In young children and infants, the headache of brain tumor at first presentation is likely to be accompanied by irritability, restlessness, crying, vomiting, dislike of having the head touched, a bulging fontanelle, head enlargement, and a cracked-pot note on skull percussion. Papilledema is uncommon in early infancy (27). In older children associated warning symptoms and signs may not be noticed until vomiting supervenes. Early, and therefore important, accompaniments of raised intracranial pressure from any cause in childhood are the psychic changes: cerebration is slowed, learning is interfered with, there may be change in personality, appearance of depression, increased fatiguability, lethargy, failure of attention, and apathy. <u>There may only be a slowing of intellectual development, rather than regression.</u> In addition, slowing of growth, and other endocrine effects can occur, and bed wetting should arouse suspicion of diabetes insipidus. Honig and Charney (49) found that 60 of 72 children with headache due to brain tumor were diagnosed within four months of onset of their headaches (42 within two months), and they considered that eleven of the remaining twelve had symptoms or signs which could have led to earlier diagnosis: these included small stature, polydipsia, alteration in character and frequency of headache, behavioral changes, blurring of vision and diplopia, incoordination.

Children with headaches should therefore be observed long enough to establish that normal physical growth and intellectual and motor development continue, that performance of all skills is maintained, and that the child shows no alteration in personality or behavior, over at least a six-month period, with occasional review thereafter. Information obtained from school reports should be included in follow-up assessment.

Pseudotumor Cerebri (benign intracranial hypertension)

Raised intracranial pressure in the absence of a space occupying lesion or of hydrocephalus is well recognized in childhood. Grant (39) reviewed 79 children aged 4 months to 14 years, and found the following associated illnesses and apparently provoking factors: middle-ear disease, tetracycline and steroid treatment, and hypocalcemia. The underlying cause(s) is not understood; possible mechanisms include increased cerebral blood volume, disturbance of intracranial venous circulation, hypersecretion of CSF (79,83).

Hydrocephalus

The more severe forms of hydrocephalus, and those associated with neural tube defect, are present in infancy, but some of the congenital and post-hemorrhagic or post-infective types may not be present until well into childhood; poor intellectual and motor performance generally predate headache in such children, but their significance may not be fully appreciated unless the large head size is noticed. In some cases, e.g., narrowing of the aqueduct of Sylvius (whether previously shunted or not) there may be periodic decompensation, and presentation with recurrent paroxysms of headache and vomiting. Others may have a more gradual build-up in pressure with low grade, chronic headache, not always obvious in very young children. It has been suggested (91) that children in whom the head size is large, either in absolute terms or relative to height, may have mild degrees of hydrocephalus manifesting only as cognitive problems; this has not been established (34).

Ocular Causes

Extraocular muscle imbalance with or without refractive error and overaccomodation can cause ocular discomfort, with headache in and around the eyes, and radiating to the frontal and temporal areas (3). The frequency of headache attributable to these causes is probably overestimated, but ophthalmic examination should always be done. The commonest findings are uncorrected hyperopia, astigmatism and convergence insufficiency; glaucoma has been described.

Sinusitis

Acute sinusitis is usually self evident, and accompanying local pain and tenderness reveals the site of infection. Headache with catarrh or chronic sinusitis (especially frontal) is more difficult to evaluate; many turn out to be of muscle tension type, in children with allergic rhinitis (7). Finally nasopharyngeal malignancy, although very rare, can occur in children.

Other Causes

Other important conditions which may present in childhood as recurrent headaches include depressive illness (63), arterial hypertension (94), pheochromocytoma, psychomotor and other forms of epilepsy (51,95) and insulinoma. The relationships between hypoglycemia and headache were discussed by Hockaday (41). Temporomandibular joint dysfunction is reported as causing head and facial pain in children, with a strong association with depression (4).

Unexplained Recurrent Headache

Most studies agree in regarding unexplained recurrent headaches in children as most likely to be migraine, or the headache of muscle tension. Psychogenic (assumed) headache is well recognized. Headache as a true conversion (hysterical) symptom also occurs. As described above, "unexplained" headache can be symptomatic of depression.

Although children with "unexplained" recurrent headaches do not have definable organic disease; their condition may be disabling, for even trivial symptoms can interfere with normal life, development, and schooling, with the possibility of long-term undesirable effects. Headache accounted for less than 1% of school absence in a recent epidemiological study (13), but also contributed to school sick bay attendance, and to time missed by leaving school early. The direct effects of headache on learning have not been studied.

Migraine

Migraine is a clinically defined disorder over- or under-diagnosed according to which of its many characteristic features are regarded as prerequisite. Epidemiological studies so far have not found good evidence that these identify a distinct syndrome (104,107). It is usually diagnosed as recurring headaches with at least two of the following three features: unilateral headache, associated nausea with or without vomiting, and focal neurological aura. This is difficult at first presentation in childhood (45), where symptoms are often overshadowed by accompanying abdominal pain or are not accurately reported, and where referral is likely to be before a recurring pattern with clear intervals is apparent. Moreover if the three criteria mentioned above are regarded as necessary, then many cases will fail to be diagnosed. Because of these difficulties, many different methods of case ascertainment have been proposed. A widely accepted approach has been that of Vahlquist (101) and Bille (5) who diagnosed migraine when headaches were paroxysmal, separated by free intervals and associated with at least two of the following four features: one sided pain, nausea, visual aura (or equivalent), family heredity (parents or siblings). Prensky and Sommer (77) required three of six features: abdominal pain, nausea or vomiting, headache confined to one side, a throbbing or pulsatile quality of the pain, complete relief after a brief period of rest, an aura (either visual, sensory or motor), and a history of migraine headaches in one or more members of the immediate family. Congdon and Forsythe (14) ascertained their large childhood series on the basis of three of the following four features: an aura, nausea, vomiting, and a family history. They observed that had they used the (stricter) criteria of Bille (5) some of their cases would have been excluded for some years.

An alternative approach for clinical purposes in children was suggested by Hockaday (44): to accept as migraine recurrent headaches that are clearly paroxysmal provided that there is return to full normal health (both mental and physical) between attacks, and that other causes of headache have been excluded. In a series of 122 childhood cases selected on this basis (43) it was found that at least two of the three chief features of migraine were present in 61% and at least one was present in a further 33%. Only 6% lacked all three features commonly held to characterize migraine (unilaterality of headache, nausea/vomiting, aura). It is recognized that the distinction between common migraine, and headache of muscle tension origin may be unclear and that, as in adults, both may occur in the same child.

Family History. The presence or absence of a family history of migraine is not helpful in diagnosis, and this is only partly because such a history is likely to be unreliable: Waters (103) found that migraine was not reported significantly more in families of migraine subjects than in families of subjects with other forms of headache or of those without headaches of any sort. The question of whether migraine is a familial disorder remains controversial (37). Lucas (64) concluded from twin studies that there is a much lower genetic factor in migraine than previously thought, and Ziegler's observations (107) from twin studies also cast doubt on a genetic component.

Prevalence. Amongst studies (mostly by self-administered questionnaire, and based on differing diagnostic criteria) in healthy groups of children, widely different migraine prevalence rates are found (Table 3). Sparks (93) found over 50% of the migraine population in schools had been to see their doctor because of headache. Even at the lowest estimate migraine is common, and this is borne out by the early age of onset described by many adults presenting with migraine. Selby and Lance (87) found 21% onset before ten years, and 25% between ten and twenty years. In a childhood series, Hockaday (43) found onset by age seven in 62% and by age ten in 86%, and Congdon and Forsythe (14) observed onset before age five in one-third of their children. Onset in infancy is well known although diagnosis is then made only retrospectively. Almost all series in younger childhood show a slightly higher incidence in boys; female preponderance arises from puberty onwards.

TABLE 3. Prevalence of Migraine* in School Children.

Authors:	Year:	Age:	Boys:	Girls:
Vahlquist	1955	10-12	4.5%	
Bille	1962	7-15	3.3%	4.4%
Dalsgaard-Nielsen et al.	1970	7-18	6.8%	7.5%
Waters	1974	10-16	9.0%	12.0%
Deubner	1977	10-15	16.0%	22.0%
Sparks**	1978	10-18	3.4%	2.5%
Sillanpaa	1983	7	2.7%	
		14	10.6%	

*Ascertained on different criteria.
**50% had consulted their doctor because of migraine.

Predisposing and Provoking Causes. Some of the immediate attack precipitants observed in childhood studies are shown in Table 4. Stress factors are prominent (66,101).

TABLE 4. Some Factors Provoking Migraine Attacks in Children.

Bille, 1962 (Ref. #5)

Stroboscopic	84%
School work	59%
Menstruation	(45%)
Conflicts, stress	33%
Physical stress	25%
Hunger	19%
Noise	19%
Motion sickness	15%
Windy weather	14%
Fatigue, uneasiness	11%
Special food, smell	8%

Congdon, Forsythe, 1979 (Ref. #14)

Traveling	9%
Cold weather	8%
Excess exercise	4%
Television	3%
Bright sunlight	2%
Certain foods	2%

Maratos, Wilkinson, 1982 (Ref. #66)

Emotional factors	86%

Head injury
(Viral encephalitis)
(Dietary factors: sensitivity, allergy)

The often stated link with menstruation is controversial. Bille (5) observed a relationship with stage of menstrual cycle in nearly 50% of post-pubertal girls, but Sparks (93) found only 21% noted a relationship between attacks and menstrual cycle stage, although 73% of girls reported having their first attack between the age of ten and fourteen years. Epstein et al. (25) also found a high incidence of migraine starting at menarche, but their study was retrospective. Waters (105) found that while headaches may begin at menarche, the majority of girls who were prepubertal were already experiencing headache. Deubner (20) also found that menarchal status was not significantly related to the presence of headache or migraine.

Frequently dietary factors are discussed; again the evidence is inadequate (61). Forsythe and Redmond (30) could find no evidence that tyramine precipitated attacks in children. A study in adults (71) reported food allergy as a cause of attacks, on the basis of dietary exclusion, subsequent food challenges and protection from challenge by cramoglycate, together with demonstration of specific IgE to certain foods by radio-allergosorbent tests. These findings have not been repeated. Merrett et al. (70) could not demonstrate any differences in total or food-specific IgE levels between dietary migraine, non-dietary migraine, and control subjects. In children Egger et al. (22) reported that the majority of a selected group with severe and unusually frequent migraine recovered when on oligo-antigenic diets (sic), and relapsed on double-blind food challenges, and that a very wide range of associated symptoms and signs were also diminished by the restriction diets. However, although 28% of the 68 children tested had high serum IgE levels, IgE antibodies did not identify the "causative" foods, and the group treated was remarkable for a high incidence of personal and familial atopy.

There is some evidence that fasting and its effects, e.g., high free fatty acid levels, may precipitate migraine (8,41,47). Pearce (75) found that migraine attacks very rarely occurred in relation to insulin induced hypoglycemia.

A minor head injury sustained, for example, in football (67) may be followed by migraine. Others have described more severe symptoms, which may be migrainous, after mild non-concussive head injury, especially in younger children. Haas et al. (40) described 50 such attacks, 40 of them occurring between ages four and fourteen years, in 25 subjects, when severe but transient neurological symptoms (hemiparesis, somnolence, irritability and vomiting, blindness or brainstem signs) followed minor head trauma after a brief latent interval.

A cellular reaction in the CSF is described in migraine, but there are also cases where viral meningitis presumably triggering the symptoms, has been diagnosed by virus isolation in patients whose clinical picture is indistinguishable from migraine of basilar, and hemiplegic, forms (11).

The possibility that migraine may be symptomatic of an underlying vascular malformation may need to be considered if the headache is always confined to the same side, if the aura is stereotyped or shows a "march" or if there are abnormal neurological signs or a cranial bruit, or if there are epileptic features. Although occasional patients diagnosed in later life as having a malformation have had headaches from early childhood, these are usually distinguishable (59), and in one large series of 500 patients presenting with headache of vascular type, no example of a vascular malformation was found (87).

Clinical Features. About 45% of boys and girls aged 10-18 studied by self-administered questionnaire in schools experienced attacks at least once monthly (93), and Congdon and Forsythe (14) observed this attack frequency in 96% of children attending a hospital pediatric clinic. Attack duration rarely exceeded ten to twelve hours in either study, and was often much shorter. Symptoms were described as severe by 37% of boys and 46% of girls (93).

In between one-third and one-half of childhood cases, migraine is of classical type. Basilar artery migraine is a well recognized form in childhood (56). In an epidemiological survey of 9059 school children aged seven to fifteen, Bille (5) observed visual aura in 50%. Congdon and Forsythe (14) found a lower incidence, 31%, but observed visceral and sensory and motor aura in a further 8% of children of all ages referred to a pediatric clinic. Hockaday (43), in a study of 122 children of all ages referred to a pediatric neurology clinic, reported very few cases with unilateral visual or sensorimotor aura (11%) but symptoms of vertebrobasilar distribution occurred in 24% (particularly in those age seven years or less), and a further 18% described an aura of unclear nature. These differences may partly reflect the ages and provenance of the cases studied.

Unusual Presentations. There are many accounts of unusual clinical presentations (Table 5) in children with migraine.

TABLE 5.   Some Special Forms of Migraine in Childhood
                 and Important Differential Diagnoses.

Some Special Forms:
          Hemiplegic (Familial)
          Ophthalmoplegic
          Prolonged stupor
          Confusional, aggressive, states
          Transient global amnesia
          Hemiballismus
          BAM with paroxysmal EEG
          Alternating hemiplegia
          Recurrent torticollis of infancy

Distinguish From:
          Sandifer syndrome
          Benign paroxysmal vertigo
          Epilepsy (epileptic cephalea, etc.)

It has been widely discussed in relation to the syndrome of alternating hemiplegia of childhood first described by Varrett and Steele (102). It is likely that some cases reported as this syndrome have migraine of vertebrobasilar type. In their review Krageloh and Aicardi (53) concluded that a distinction should be made between children with onset of the alternating hemiplegia syndrome in infancy, who may show permanent and sometimes progressive neurological abnormality, and where the pathogenesis is unknown, and cases of later onset where a diagnosis of migraine may well be appropriate. The distinction is important in view of a recent report of effective therapy with flunarizine. Migraine has been described presenting in children as an acute confusional state (23,24,31), prolonged stupor (58) and transient global amnesia (52). Other special forms are better recognized, e.g., hemiplegic migraine (54), familial hemiplegic migraine (35), the Alice in Wonderland syndrome (36), ophthalmoplegic migraine (81) which must be distinguished from the painful ophthalmoplegia of the Tolosa-Hunt syndrome recorded in early childhood by Terrence and Samaha in 1973 (98).

Possible Associations. It is often stated that some childhood complaints, e.g., cyclical vomiting, the periodic syndrome, abdominal migraine (sic), recurrent abdominal pain syndrome, may represent "equivalents" of migraine as usually defined. The links are not established, one difficulty being that many of the disorders considered are ill defined, not easily distinguishable, and therefore difficult to study in an epidemiological sense. It is generally held that most recurrent abdominal pain syndromes are psychogenically determined (16,73), although this may be difficult to establish (68). Congdon and Forsythe (14) found their incidence very low in a large series of childhood migraine, where only 3% gave an account of abdominal pain attacks before headache attacks started. Christensen and Mortensen (12) found an increased incidence of abdominal pain syndromes in children of parents who were still experiencing abdominal symptoms, but not in those whose parents gave only a past history of childhood episodes. Deubner (20) in an epidemiological study did not find a significant association between migraine and cyclic or nervous vomiting, nor between migraine and abdominal pain as recalled by children aged 10 to 15 (although as recounted by their parents, there was a strong association); he concluded that his findings contradicted the idea "that migraine is a member of a family of periodic disorders".

An association between migraine and somnambulism was reported by Barabas et al. (1) on the basis that the (proposed) relationship might reflect serotonin "instability". Bille (5) did not find an association with somnambulism, but reported a high incidence of other sleep disorders.

It is sometimes suggested that benign paroxysmal vertigo is a form of migraine in childhood. Vertigo is well known as a symptom during the aura phase of migraine (26), suggesting brainstem, or temporal lobe involvement, but the syndrome described by Basser (2) is clinically, and on natural history, very different, and it is in most cases associated with vestibular nerve abnormality (21), when it is clearly distinguished from migraine. A relationship between benign paroxysmal torticollis of infancy and migraine appears possible (19). The Sandifer syndrome should be distinguished (106).

Much has been written about the relationship between migraine and epilepsy. There are many reports of a greater than chance association between these common disorders, but they are in patients selected by hospital or clinical referral. There is no epidemiological evidence that migraine and constitutional epilepsy are related. Neither Bille's population study in school children (5), nor the very large prospective study of Lance and Anthony (55) showed any link. Similarly there is little evidence that frequent, long-standing, severe, or complicated migraine leads to the appearance of epilepsy, or of paroxysmal EEG change, in previously non-epileptic subjects (15,42,46,82,108), except in rare instances (69,76,90).

Alteration, or loss, of consciousness occur not uncommonly during the course of migraine attacks, in relation to syncope, or to postulated brainstem reticular formation involvement (60). Occasionally convulsive features occur as well. Electroencephalographic abnormalities, sometimes paroxysmal, occurring transiently with attacks or as a continuous feature, are described in relation to vertebrobasilar migraine (10,57,96). All these clinical and EEG features have, according to circumstances, been interpreted as effects of migraine in a normal subject, or in one who is potentially epileptic by reason of constitutional tendency or (rarely) because of organic disease (76,90). Further diagnostic difficulty between migraine and epilepsy arises particularly in some of the less common presentations (v.s.) of childhood migraine, such as acute confusional states, and prolonged stupor, or some of the examples of so-called alternating hemiplegia in older children. Conversely, the headache symptoms which are sometimes prominent in children with temporal lobe epilepsy, or post-ictally, and so-called seizure headaches (51,95), sometimes lead to diagnostic difficulty.

Prognosis. Childhood migraine is generally held to have a good prognosis, but this may not be so, although long remissions do occur. Bille (6) found 34% of children free from attacks six years after first ascertainment, and 41% free at 16 years of follow-up; by age 30 years or more, however, 60% of the series were still having attacks although many had been free for a period in their second or third decade. Hockaday (42) observed remissions as long as ten years, followed by recurrence; the same study found that males outgrew their attacks more often than females and that basilar artery migraine was more likely to stop than either common migraine, or migraine with unilateral aura. Sillanpaa (88) reported that migraine starting before age eight improved or ceased by age 14 in 58% of cases, although the later outcome in this epidemiological study is not yet known.

Management. Accurate diagnosis, well founded reassurance, and careful enquiry and advice about predisposing and provoking causes, are as important in children as in adults. A school report is often most helpful in elucidating psychogenic and other factors, such as teasing, bullying, learning difficulties, television, minor head trauma, excessive exercise. Stress factors may be difficult to identify, e.g., when a child is subject to abuse (verbal or physical) or deprivation within the family.

In the acute attack, treatment should if possible be limited to the administration of mild, easily soluble analgesic drugs (aspirin, paracetamol) early in the attack, together with a short rest and a high calorie drink. If nausea or vomiting is prominent, then anti-emetics may be given, orally or parenterally. Prochlorperazine and metoclopramide (taken 20 minutes before an analgesic) are widely used, although the latter in particular carries the risk of severe extrapyramidal reactions in children, even after brief administration (32). Ergotamine preparations, whose benefit is questionable (99), should be used in low dosage, and avoided altogether in young children. Propranolol has been recommended for treatment of the acute attack (100). There is no place for the use of strong analgesic drugs; if symptoms are severe, a parenteral sedative is preferable.

General advice and adequate treatment for each attack as it occurs are adequate for most children. Prophylactic treatment is recommended only when attacks continue to be so frequent, or so severe, as to be disabling, or in the rare cases where there is a dense neurological deficit in the aura phase. It is difficult to find a prophylactic drug of established value in children. Sills et al. (89) found clonidine ineffective. Propranolol was found effective in one study in childhood (65), but not in a recent double-blind controlled trial (29). Forsythe has also found pizotifen ineffective in a double-blind controlled study (personal communication). Prophylaxis with aspirin (74) is sometimes recommended although there is as yet no published study of its use in children. A recent double-blind study found flunarizine helpful in children (92). The mild sedative action of some antihistamines, or the diazepines, is often beneficial, but these remedies should be used only briefly, to try to "break" an established rhythm of recurrent attack. Because of their adverse effects on cerebral function and development, anticonvulsant drugs should be used only in children who experience both migraine and epilepsy, or tried in children with paroxysmal EEG abnormalities. Other measures such as restriction diets (22), acupuncture (63), biofeedback, autohypnosis and psychotherapy (48) have not been adequately evaluated. Restriction diet treatment is very difficult to maintain, and other maneuvers are not suitable for younger children.

Most children respond to reassurance, general advice, and simple remedies given for attacks as they arise. All management must be aimed at allowing the child to live with his disorder. Because most children with migraine do respond to treatment, or show a natural remission, failure to respond should be regarded as an indication to reconsider the diagnosis.

Tension Headache

Headache due to cervical and scalp muscle tension resulting from anxiety is rare in very young children, but can occur in middle childhood years, and is common in older children and juveniles. Distinction from migraine can be difficult; and, as in adults, migraine and tension headache may occur together. The clinical features are as in adults. Children with tension headache may appear pale, and are often anorexic, but rarely vomit. There may or may not be interference with ordinary activities. Mild analgesics are sometimes helpful.

Other Unexplained Headache

Psychogenic (assumed) headache is quite a common symptom, which needs to be distinguished from genuine headache; the reason for it should be determined wherever possible. School refusal is an important cause.

Headache occurring apparently as a conversion symptom in children is not adequately described, but it is a clinically important diagnosis, needing urgent psychiatric management. The youngest personally observed case was age nine years. The selective nature of the limitation of activity, and the disability, is striking.

REFERENCES

1. Barabas, G., Ferrari, M., and Matthews, W. S. (1983): Neurology, 33:948.
2. Basser, L. S. (1964): Brain, 87:141.
3. Behrens, M. M. (1978): Med. Clin. N. Amer., 62:507.
4. Belfer, M. L., and Kaban, L. B. (1982): Pediatrics, 69:564.
5. Bille, B. (1962): Acta Paediatrica, 51:1 (Suppl. 136).
6. Bille, B. (1982): Panminerva Medica – Europa Medica, 24:57.
7. Birt, D. (1978): Med. Clin. N. Amer., 62:523.
8. Blau, J. N., and Cumings, J. N. (1966): Brit. Med. J., 2:1242.
9. Brewis, M., Poskanzer, D. C., and Rolland, C. (1966): Acta Neurol. Scandinav., 42:1 (Suppl. 24).
10. Camfield, P. R., Metrakos, K., and Andermann, F. (1978): Neurology, 28:584.
11. Casteels-Van Daele, M., Standaert, L., Boel, M., Smeets, E., Colaert, J., and Desmyter, J. (1981): Lancet, 1:1366.
12. Christensen, M. F., and Mortensen, O. (1975): Arch. Dis. Childh., 50:110.
13. Collin, C., Hockaday, J. M., and Waters, W. E. (1984): Submitted for publication.
14. Congdon, P. J.; and Forsythe, W. I. (1979): Develop. Med. Child Neurol., 21:209.
15. Connor, R. C. R. (1962): Lancet, 2:1072.
16. Coulthard, M. (1984): Arch. Dis. Childh., 59:189.
17. Dalessio, D. J. (1980): In: Headache and Other Head Pain, 4th Edition, edited by H. G. Wolff. Oxford University Press, London.
18. Dalsgaard-Nielsen, T., Engberg-Pedersen, H., and Holm, H. E. (1970): Danish Med. Bull., 17:138.
19. Deonna, T., and Martin, D. (1981): Arch. Dis. Childh., 56:956.
20. Deubner, D. C. (1977): Headache, 17:173.
21. Dunn, D. W., and Snyder, C. H. (1976): Amer. J. Dis. Children, 130:1099.
22. Egger, J., Carter, C. M., Wilson, J., Turner, M. W., and Soothill, J. F. (1983): Lancet, 2:865.
23. Ehyai, A., and Fenichel, G. M. (1978): Arch. Neurol., 35:368.
24. Emery, E. S. (1977): Pediatrics, 60:110.
25. Epstein, M. T., Hockaday, J. M., and Hockaday, T. D. R. (1975): Lancet, 1:543.
26. Eviatar, L., and Eviatar, A. (1977): Pediatrics, 59:833.
27. Farwell, J. R., and Dohrmann, G. J. (1978): Arch. Neurol., 35:533.
28. Fitzsimons, J. M. (1963): Tubercle, 44:87.
29. Forsythe, I., Gillies, D., and Sills, M. (1984): Develop. Med. Child Neurol.
30. Forsythe, W. I., and Redmond, A. (1974): Develop. Med. Child Neurol., 16:794.

31. Gascon, G., and Barlow, C. (1970): Pediatrics, 45:628.
32. Gatrad, A. R. (1976): Develop. Med. Child Neurol., 18:767.
33. Geissinger, J. D., and Bucy, P. C. (1971): Arch. Neurol., 24:125.
34. Gillberg, C., and Rasmussen, P. (1983): Develop. Med. Child Neurol., 24:198.
35. Glista, G. G., Millinger, J. F., and Rooke, E. D. (1975): Mayo Clinic Proc., 50:307.
36. Golden, G. S. (1979): Pediatrics, 63:517.
37. Goldstein, M., and Chen, T. C. (1982): In: Headache: Physiopathological and Clinical Concepts, Advances in Neurology, Volume 33, edited by M. Critchley, A. P. Friedman, S. Gorini, and F. Sicuteri, pp. 377–390. Raven Press, New York.
38. Gordon, N. (1977): Develop. Med. Child Neurol., 19:540.
39. Grant, D. N. (1971): Arch. Dis. Childh., 46:651.
40. Haas, D. C., Pineda, G. S., and Lourie, H. (1975): Arch. Neurol., 32:727.
41. Hockaday, J. M. (1975): In: Modern Topics in Medicine, edited by J. Pearce, pp. 124–137. William Heinemann Medical Books, Ltd., London.
42. Hockaday, J. M. (1978): In: Current Concepts in Migraine Research, edited by R. Greene, pp. 41–48. Raven Press, New York.
43. Hockaday, J. M. (1979): Develop. Med. Child Neurol., 21:455.
44. Hockaday, J. M. (1982): Brit. J. Hosp. Med., 27:383.
45. Hockaday, J. M. (1984): In: Progress in Child Health, Vol. 1, edited by J. A. Macfarlane, pp. 13–24. Churchill-Livingstone, Edinburgh.
46. Hockaday, J. M., and Whitty, C. W. M. (1969): Brain, 92:769.
47. Hockaday, J. M., Williamson, D. H., and Whitty, C. W. M. (1971): Lancet, 1:1153.
48. Hoelsher, T. J., and Lichstein, K. L. (1984): Headache, 24:94.
49. Honig, P. J., and Charney, E. B. (1982): Amer. J. Dis. Children, 136:121.
50. Idriss, Z. H., Gutman, L. T., and Kronfol, N. M. (1978): Clin. Pediatr., 17:738.
51. Isler, H., Wieser, H. G., and Egli, M. (1984): In, Progress in Migraine Research, Volume 2, edited by F. C. Rose, pp. 69–82. Pitman Publ., London.
52. Jensen, T. S. (1980): Develop. Med. Child Neurol., 22:654.
53. Krageloh, I., and Aicardi, J. (1980): Develop. Med. Child Neurol., 22:784.
54. Lai, C., Ziegler, D. K., Lansky, L. L., and Torres, F. (1982): J. Pediatr., 101:696.
55. Lance, J. W., and Anthony, M. (1966): Arch. Neurol., 15:536.
56. Lapkin, M. L., and Golden, G. S. (1978): Amer. J. Dis. Children, 132:278.

57. Lapkin, M. L., French, J. F., Golden, G. S., and Rowan, A. J. (1977): Neurology, 27:580.
58. Lee, C. H., and Lance, J. W. (1977): Headache, 17:32.
59. Lees, F. (1962): J. Neurol. Neurosurg. Psychiat., 25:45.
60. Lees, F., and Watkins, S. M. (1963): Lancet, 2:647.
61. Leviton, A. (1984): Develop. Med. Child Neurol., 26:542.
62. Ling, W., Oftedal, T. G., and Weinberg, W. (1970): Amer. J. Dis. Child., 120:122.
63. Loh, L., Nathan, P. W., Schott, G. D., and Zilkha, K. J. (1984): J. Neurol. Neurosurg. Psychiat., 47:333.
64. Lucas, R. N. (1977): J. Psychosomat. Res., 20:147.
65. Ludvigsson, J. (1973): Lancet, 2:799.
66. Maratos, J., and Wilkinson, M. (1982): Cephalagia, 2:179.
67. Matthews, W. B. (1972): Brit. Med. J., 2:326.
68. McGrath, P. J., Goodman, J. T., Firestone, P., Shipman, R., and Peters, S. (1983): Arch. Dis. Childh., 58:888.
69. Ment, L. R., Duncan, C. D., Parcells, P. R., and Collins, W. F. (1980): Child's Brain, 7:261.
70. Merrett, J., Peatfield, R. C., Rose, F. C., and Merrett, T. G. (1983): J. Neurol. Neurosurg. Psychiat., 46:738.
71. Monro, J., Brostoff, J., Carini, C., and Zilkha, K. (1980): Lancet, 2:1.
72. Naughten, E., Newton, R., Weindling, A. M., and Bower, B. D. (1981): Lancet, 2:973.
73. Nicol, A. R. (1982): Brit. J. Hosp. Med., 27:351.
74. O'Neill, B. P., and Mann, J. D. (1978): Lancet, 2:1179.
75. Pearce, J. (1971): J. Neurol. Neurosurg. Psychiat., 34:154.
76. Pearce, J. M. S., and Foster, J. B. (1965): Neurology, 15:333.
77. Prensky, A. L., and Sommer, D. (1979): Neurology, 29:506.
78. Registrar General's Annual Report, (1978): Mortality Statistics. HMSO, London.
79. Reid, A. C., Matheson, M. S., and Teasdale, G. (1980): Lancet, 2:7.
80. Roberton, M., Barbor, P., and Hull, D. (1982): Brit. Med. J., 285:1399.
81. Robertson, W. C., and Schnitzler, E. R. (1978): Pediatrics, 61:886.
82. Rossi, L. N., Mumenthaler, M., and Vassella, F. (1980): Neuropediatrics, 11:27.
83. Rush, J. A. (1983): Brit. J. Hosp. Med., 29:320.
84. Rushton, J. G., and Rooke, E. D. (1962): Headache, 2:147.
85. Schulte, F. J. (1984): Neuropediatrics, 15:3.
86. Sedzimer, C. B., and Robinson, J. (1973): J. Neurosurg., 38:269.
87. Selby, G., and Lance, J. W. (1960): J. Neurol. Neurosurg. Psychiat., 23:23.
88. Sillanpaa, M. (1983): Headache, 23:15.
89. Sills, M., Congdon, P., and Forsythe, I. (1982): Develop. Med. Child Neurol., 24:837.
90. Slatter, K. H. (1968): Brain, 91:85.
91. Smith, R. (1981): Develop. Med. Child Neurol., 23:626.

92. Sorge, F., De Simone, R., Marano, E., Orefice, G., and Carrieri, P. (1985): Proceedings of 2nd International Headache Society. Copenhagen.
93. Sparks, J. P. (1978): Practitioner, 221:407.
94. Still, J. L., and Cottom, D. (1967): Arch. Dis. Childh., 42:34.
95. Swaiman, K. F., and Frank, Y. (1978): Develop. Med. Child Neurol., 20:580.
96. Swanson, J. W., and Vick, N. A. (1978): Neurology, 28:782.
97. Swartz, M. N., and Dodge, P. R. (1965): New Engl. J. Med., 272:725-730 and 779-787.
98. Terrence, C. F., and Samaha, F. J. (1973): Develop. Med. Child Neurol., 15:506.
99. Thrush, D. (1984): In: Dilemmas in the Management of the Neurological Patient, edited by C. Warlow and J. Garfield, pp. 106-114. Churchill-Livingstone, Edinburgh.
100. Tokola, R., and Hokkanen, E. (1978): Brit. Med. J., 2:1098.
101. Vahlquist, B. (1955): Internat. Arch. Allergy, 7:348.
102. Varrett, S., and Steele, J. C. (1971): Pediatrics, 47:675.
103. Waters, W. E. (1971): Brit. Med. J., 2:77.
104. Waters, W. E. (1973): Internat. J. Epidemiol., 2:189.
105. Waters, W. E. (1974): The Epidemiology of Migraine. Boehringer-Ingelheim, Bracknell Berkshire, England.
106. Werlin, S. L., D'Souza, B. J., Hogan, W. J., Dodds, W. J., and Arndorfer, R. C. (1980): Develop. Med. Child Neurol., 22:374.
107. Ziegler, D. K. (1978): Res. Clin. Stud. Headache, 5:21.
108. Ziegler, D. K. (1984): In: Progress in Migraine Research, Volume 2, edited by F. C. Rose, pp. 1-8. Pitman Publ., London.

The Management of Headache, edited by F. Clifford Rose. Raven Press, New York © 1988.

FUTURE PERSPECTIVES

Otto Appenzeller, MD, PhD

Professor of Neurology and Medicine,
University of New Mexico School of Medicine,
Albuquerque, New Mexico 87131, U.S.A.

Headache is a frequent symptom and can be the manifestation of a variety of diseases. The future of headache research and of innovative management discussed in this Chapter refers to the vast majority of patients who have no discernible intracranial lesion to account for their headache. This includes vascular headaches of the migrainous type, scalp muscle contraction headache, and post-traumatic headache.

The nature of these common headaches has been the subject of investigation for decades, but all attempts at unravelling their pathogenesis have so far been unsuccessful. Although a number of proposals have been made which explain some, but not all, features of vascular, scalp muscle contraction, and post-traumatic headaches, a personal bias invariably enters into the prediction of future trends and what follows is no exception.

A number of triggrs reliably reproduce in some individuals their usual spontaneous headaches, and these induced headache attacks offer an opportunity to search for clues on pathogenesis and for new therapies.

Barogenic Headache

Headache can be reliably reproduced in some migraineurs with changes in barometric pressure. Such headaches, though more often vascular in nature, are sometimes of scalp muscle contraction type. They are important in ascent to high altitudes where ambient gas pressures affect living things, and in depth dives where increasing pressure similarly influences a variety of body functions.

The commonest manifestation of maladapted sojourners who arrive at an altitude of about 2,500 m is acute mountain sickness (AMS), the most disabling clinical manifestation of which is severe and often pounding headache. Nausea, dimmed vision, restlessness, palpitation, anorexia, sleeplessness, and anxiety also occur. During altitude exposure, there is an increase in vascular permeability which is clinically manifest by retinopathy, increased intraocular pressure, and cerebral and visceral edema. Hypoxia is always associated with high altitude illness and the concomitant low barometric pressure may also be of importance. This is suggested by the delay in onset of clinical manifestations of about six to 96 hours after arrival at high altitude so that secondary or tertiary influences may be triggers of AMS and its headache. While fluid retention is universal in all individuals, this occurs in a setting of increased sodium excretion, but patients with AMS have less sodium excretion than those not affected by the illness.

The cerebral edema of high altitude is indistinguishable clinically or pathologically from that occurring at sea level, but measurement of cerebral metabolism up to an altitude of 5,500 m has not disclosed measurable changes, and acclimatized mountaineers have no difficulty in record keeping and meteorologic data collection in the Himalayas when finally acclimatized, though some cerebral edema persists in such individuals. The neuropsychologic effects of high altitude, however, are similar to those found in mild alcohol intoxication. The visual system is affected and the increase in intraocular pressure may contribute to the headache, which is exercise sensitive. Focal neurologic deficits at high altitude include tetraparesis and drop attacks, which have been attributed to falls in vertebral artery bloodflow. At rest, measurement of cerebral blood flow, both acutely and after acclimatization, have shown considerable increase in cerebral blood flow using the nitrous oxide method (23) and longitudinal studies of carotid artery flow using Doppler techniques have confirmed an increase in common carotid and preauricular artery flow related to altitude (5).

Migraine and cluster headache are precipitated by altitude exposure, but the relation of the change in barometric pressure or hypoxia to the genesis of headaches is not clear. The increase in cerebral blood flow suggests that the initial vasoconstriction so characteristic of migrainous attacks does not occur at high altitude, yet the aura of migraine can regularly be induced in some individuals by specific altitude exposure, but without subsequent headache. This supports the idea that migraine might be initiated by abnormal neurogenic discharges rather than primary vascular dysfunction (7), the hypoxia being the trigger and the changes in blood flow merely secondary manifestations of neurogenic dysfunction.

AMS, including its headache, is related to the speed of ascent and inversely related to age, and the time taken for acclimatization. Endurance training is protective and facilitates adaptation to altitude, presumably by increasing maximum oxygen consumption. While the headache of acute mountain sickness varies in its intensity and characteristics between individuals, there is little variation on altitude exposure in AMS in the same subject, a close replication of previous illness on subsequent attempts at altitude sojourn being the rule. An inherent characteristic of the headache and other features of AMS is an individual response to altitude exposure.

Effort migraine is also more frequent at altitude. Coital headache may make its initial appearance with relatively moderate altitude exposure and may persist after return to sea level for prolonged periods of time. The cerebrospinal fluid pressure increases in AMS and evidence of cerebral edema on biopsy of mountaineers has been found (24).

Changes in body water, endocrine secretion and vasoconstriction in a variety of vascular beds occur. The administration of glucose improves altitude headache and hypoglycemia is known to be associated with migrainous attacks at sea level. Acute mountain sickness is worsened by alcohol, and migraine at sea level can be triggered by alcohol. All these support a similar primary neurogenic cause of altitude headache and of migraine.

Difficulties arise in explaining some clinical features. The early vascular component of altitude headache occurs in association with increasing intracranial pressure. Blood flow in the carotid increases and retinal artery vasodilatation has been demonstrated. If the retinal circulation reflects the circulation in the brain, then the cerebral edema may be caused by increasing filtration through the parenchymal microcirculation. Another explanation may be that the early throbbing component of altitude headache causes an increase in flow through functionally activated arteriovenous anastomoses, and the brain edema may be primary in response to the hypoxia and then trigger the vascular component of the headache, which is secondary, and the result of neurogenic vasodilatation of only part of the cerebral circulation. Whatever the eventual explanation for the pathogenesis of altitude headache might be, it will have important bearing on the management of vascular headaches at sea level.

Altitude and Toothache

Rapid ascent to high altitude was found to be associated in pilots with pain in teeth and in the maxillary antrum. The painful teeth were those that had been traumatized in the past, even years earlier, by dental work. Such pilots, if subjected to needle pricks to the nasal mucosa near the ostium of the maxillary sinus, were found to have pain at the site of the needle pricks and in the teeth previously subjected to trauma. Experiments were carried out with teeth filled under general anesthesia. After recovery from the anesthetic, pain was elicited after stimulation of the nasal mucous membrane in the appropriate teeth, but if the teeth were filled under local anesthesia, stimulation by needle pricks of the nasal mucosa no longer induced pain in the teeth. When these experiments were carried out, it was thought that this type of pain had some bearing on long-lasting or even permanent changes in the nervous system resulting from a "memory for pain" in the periphery.

These clinical experiments might have some bearing on the genesis of chronic pain syndromes and particularly on atypical facial pain. Pain in teeth and migraine with altitude exposure suggests also that study of the pathogenesis of this "peripheral memory for pain" might have bearing on "status migrainosus" and "chronic cranial cephalalgia."

Headache and Diving

Skip breathing is employed by many divers. Anecdotal reports claim that this technique causes headache, but increasing experience and repeated skip breathing diminish this headache which may completely disappear. Inexperienced divers, it is claimed, who skip breathe, have an unusual sensitivity of cerebral arteries to an increase in carbon dioxide level. This increased sensitivity decreases with diving experience, but the headache may recur at depth with unusual exertion, because of increase in CO_2 levels due to faster production associated with muscular contraction.

Pain in the sinuses is also common. It is accentuated in those divers with cold sensitivity or allergic conditions which may cause swelling of the mucous membranes and block the ostia of the sinuses. When using scuba gear, the expansion of air from the high pressure tank to the lower pressure of the surrounding water results in cooling of the air. This cold air passes across the sinus mucous membranes causing pain which may be similar to that of "ice cream" headache.

The cavities in teeth may also cause pain in divers, and this has been attributed to expansion of gas pockets which stimulate nociceptive afferents from the teeth and result in severe ache and pain, which may persist well after the dive.

Muscle contraction headache can be produced in susceptible divers by a tightening grip of the mouthpiece between the teeth. Conscious relaxation during prolonged scuba dives is helpful. This supports the contention that scalp muscle contraction headaches are associated with an increase in spindle afferent activity from the muscles of mastication (2).

Migraine-like symptoms during hyperbaric compression occur repeatedly in susceptible individuals, scotomas and headache being frequent in those with a past history of migraine.

The platelet count decreases and clumping of platelet increases after depth dives. The similarity of platelet changes in dives and in migraineurs may point to some important common pathogenetic mechanisms. Moreover, stress related changes in creatine phosphokinase, alkaline phosphatase, aspartate amino transferase, cortisol, and free fatty acids, have all been found in divers. Many of these changes in blood constituents have not been investigated, but some parallel those found in migraineurs.

Exercise and Headache

Effort migraine is indistinguishable from attacks occurring without exertion. It is characterized, like ordinary attacks, by scotomata, nausea, and pulsatile, severe, usually retroorbital, unilateral pain, but its duration is often shorter than ordinary migrainous attacks. It can occur with repeated effort and sometimes only part of the migrainous syndrome is reproduced, e.g., without the headache.

Effort migraine may rarely be associated with transient or permanent neurologic deficits, particularly if the exercise is unaccustomed, carried out at altitude, accompanied by alcohol intake, or hypoglycemia. The similarity between known triggers of migraine offers an opportunity for further investigation of the neurogenic components of migraine and modification of these by training.

Prolonged low level effort in poorly trained individuals is also associated with vascular headache. Like ordinary migraine, hypoglycemia, dehydration, excessive heatloads and altitude may promote this type of vascular headache. Because focal neurologic deficits do not occur, this headahce may serve as a model for common rather than classic migraine.

A third type of exertional headache occurs at any level of physical activity, frequently in untrained individuals and in overconfident exercisers. It is an occipital throbbing pain accompanied by nausea; no neurologic dysfunction is found. It increases with increasing effort, and persists for hours after exertion. Support of neck muscles, analgesics taken before exertion, and endurance training all tend to prevent recurrences. This type of pain may serve as a model for combined headache.

Hypotheses abound on the mechanisms of the beneficial effects of endurance training on vascular headache. One favored view is that the decreased sympathetic tone of endurance-trained athletes (evidenced by resting bradycardia), probably the result of central rather than peripheral alterations in nervous system function, explains its usefulness in therapy. This is supported by some clinical findings, but requires more evidence before it can be generally accepted.

Vascular Headache and Epilepsy

The relationship between these forms of central nervous system dysfunction has been a matter of conjecture for decades.

Kindling, definitely shown only in animals, depends in part on the integrity of the substantia nigra. Clinical studies have demonstrated an absence of epilepsy in patients with Parkinson's disease.

The autonomic discharge accompanying cluster headache might arise in the brainstem close to the substantia nigra, and we have seen patients who had a see-saw relationship between cluster attacks and fits which were mutually exclusive (3).

Epilepsy is rare if not entirely absent in large cluster headache populations (15). Further search for clinically useful hints by epidemiologic techniques might yield information about epilepsy, vascular headache, and the episodic nervous system dysfunction which underlies these disorders.

Minor Trauma and Migraine

Soccer players who head the ball, professional boxers, and others who may sustain minor head injury, may develop repeated typical attacks of migraine. The pathogenesis of this type of migraine is unknown, but the occasional recurrence of "second impact catastrophic headache" should not be forgotten. A peculiar unexplained susceptibility to disastrous brain edema after sequential minor head impacts does exist. The proposal has been made that a loss of vasomotor tone causes the fatal increase in intracranial pressure in these rare cases, but the initial injury to the nervous system supports the neurogenic origin of this dangerous vascular complication.

Hormones and Headache

Vascular headaches occur more often among all contraceptive users and withdrawal of birth control pills produces improvement. Remission of migraine during the third trimester of pregnancy is also common. A relationship between estrogen and the vasomotor system has been proposed and prolonged elevated estrodial levels are assocaited with excessive reactivity of cranial vessels when estrogen levels drop (27). Women with menstrual migraine are more likely to have migraine onset at menarche. They often have the premenstrual syndrome and also show improvement in their migraine during pregnancy. Hormone levels (plasma estrogen and progesterone) are significantly higher in such women when compared to non-menstrual migraineurs and non-migrainous women (10). Examination of endometrial biopsies from women with menstrual migraine often shows abnormal arterioles, and similar morphologic changes are associated with an increased incidence of headache during oral contraceptive use (12). The pathogenetic role of monoamines in migraine, as in the behavioral changes which accompany attacks of migraine, is not clear. Serotonin and noradrenaline, which have been implicated in the genesis of migraine, are known to be important in controlling blood vessel reactivity. Oral contraceptive use increases cortisol release and this has been attributed to an increased turnover of tryptophan (20). The pill-associated depression and migraine has tentatively been attributed to a decrease in brain serotonin in patients who are on birth control pills, and this has been implicated in the genesis of some migrainous attacks (1). Examination of endometrial monoamine oxidase content in those on estrogen and progesterone has shown increases in the levels of this enzyme in endometrial glands, and similar changes have been postulated to occur in the brain of migraineurs who take birth control pills. If an increase in monoamine oxidase occurs in the brain, it might increase serotonin and other vasoactive amine turnover and thus cause low amine levels favoring depression and migraine.

Evidence that the immune system and the brain communicate with each other through neurotransmitters, hormones, and nerves has been presented. During the immune response, the brain receives messages from immunologic cells which modify brain activity through the release of histamine, serotonin, prostaglandins, and interferon, some of which share amino acid sequences with ACTH and beta-endorphin (25). The brain, in turn, influences the immune system and learned histamine release has recently been demonstrated (21).

Experimentally, a remarkable reduction has been found in serotonin-fluorescent mast cells associated with uterine vessels in progesterone and combined estrogen-progesterone treated animals. In addition, such animals have an increased number of mast cells in association with cerebral vessels. Noradrenaline in perivascular adrenergic nerves and myometrial blood vessels of estrogen-treated and combined estrogen-progesterone-treated rats were similarly reduced (22). The changes in uterine and cerebral vessels of experimental animals may give a clue to the pathogenesis of menstrual and oral contraceptive-associated migraine. Mast cells not only contain histamine and other vasoactive substances but also participate in the immune response. Activation of the immune system is thought to be important in some types of vascular headaches, and this, in turn, might exert effects through monoamines which are influenced by changing levels of sex hormones and by other neurotransmitters. The progesterone-induced experimental intracranial perivascular mastocytosis might provide a model for hormone-associated migraine and for the testing of future antimigrainous drugs in animals.

Headache Associated with Disease in Other Systems

Headache may be a frequent accompaniment of diseases in other systems. An example is the occurrence of vascular headache of the migrainous type in patients with non-specific inflammatory disease of the bowel. Examination of resected specimens in such individuals showed large numbers of mast cells infiltrating the diseased part of the gut. The role of mast cells in the genesis of migraine remains hypothetical, but offers a fruitful avenue for further investigation.

Vascular headache is a common feature in autoerythrocyte sensitization syndrome, occurring in 60% of patients. This syndrome, also known as psychogenic purpura or the Gardner-Diamond syndrome, is characterized by recurrent spontaneous painful bruising and often mucosal bleeding. The severe and frequent vascular headache that is part of the illness can be accompanied by ocular pain, scotomata, stiff neck, nausea, vomiting and, in one of three recently examined cases, ipsilateral pupillary dilatation, increased sweating, and boggy periorbital bruising. Other neurologic symptoms reported in this syndrome include syncope, paresthesia, transient paresis, and less commonly, sensory changes, tremor, aphasia, seizures, and ataxia (19). Approximately 100 patients with this syndrome have been reported, but no consistent laboratory abnormalities have been found. A granular pattern of immune complex deposition was demonstrated in glomerular basement membranes in some patients, and the antigen has been identified as erythrocyte stroma (18). Decreased complement, elevated IgG and IgM, and B and T cell abnormalities have been described (14). Such patients have frequent psychologic abnormalities characterized by hysteria, masochism, depression, anxiety, and an inability to deal with hostile feelings (19). Explanations for this peculiar syndrome have been, as with migraine, both immunologic and psychogenic, but the vascular headache frequently found in this disorder has remained enigmatic. Support for the immunologic pathogenesis of the disease has come from the finding that intradermal injection of autologous washed red cells in some, but not all, patients produces bruising. The frequently grotesque psychologic abnormalities which have been described argue for a psychogenic etiology, including self injury. No effective curative treatment for the bruising nor for the headache has been found, and the disease is prolonged and intractable.

Neurotensin, substance P, and VIP have been demonstrated in normal cutaneous, and perivascular, nerves and in sweat glands (13). These substances are important in the inflammatory response. Intravenous neurotensin causes blood vessel dilatation which can be abolished by the administration of H_1 receptor blockers (9). Neurotensin binding sites have been identified on mast cells and it is the most potent mast cell degranulator known to date (11). Neurotensin modulates the inflammatory response through its effect on substance P and decreased neurotensin enhances inflammation.

Skin biopsies of spontaneous bruises in some patients with this syndrome may show perivascular mast cell infiltrates. Because of this, the histochemical examination of skin specimens for neurotensin, substance P, and other neuropeptides may shed light on the genesis of headache, not only in autoerythrocyte sensitization, but also in other vascular headaches where increase in mast cells in temple skin have been demonstrated (4,17).

Immunohistochemistry in Vascular Headache

Vasodilatation of extracranial vessels is an important component of migraine and cluster headache. The mechanism for this sometimes focal vasodilatation is not clear. Immunohistochemical techniques can be used to demonstrate neuropeptides and other substances in nerve fibers. Temple skin biopsies from patients with migraine and cluster headache have been carried out and examined for clues to mechanisms of vasodilatation using this technique.

Noradrenergic and serotoninergic nerve fibers, and neuropeptide-containing nerve profiles in patients with cluster headache were compared with migraineurs. An increase in substance P and in mast cells, particularly on the headache side, was found in cluster patients. Substance P is a potent vasodilator and also has a pivotal role in the flare component of the triple response (16). This supports the proposal that axonal reflexes might be important in the genesis of unilateral pain in cluster attacks. Serotonin was present only in cluster headache skin. The possibility that repeated axonal reflex activation causes proliferation of both serotonin and substance P containing fibers in the skin must be considered.

These results may have clinical significance. Potential useful peptide analogues have recently been manufactured. Substance P antagonists, in a number of peripheral tissues, have revealed the functional significance of this peptide in peripheral nerves. Peripheral vasodilatation evoked by antidromic stimulation of sensory nerves (axonal reflex) can be antagonized by new pharmaceutical preparations which might therefore offer different approaches to cluster headache treatment.

Possible New Approaches to the Pharmacotherapy of Headache

The interest in ergot research has a history dating back to 1875. In the early part of this century Dale described the usefulness of ergotoxine. Since then, a number of derivatives of the original ergot compounds have proved useful in headache and other conditions; one example is bromocriptine. Research on ergotamine compounds continues unabated in spite of the success of already available ergotamines. The main thrust of studies is concentrated on different receptor sites, agonists and antagonists of ergot and on ergotamine receptors which may be predominantly noradrenergic, serotoninergic, or dopaminergic. Knowledge in these areas will spur pharmaceutical companies to produce agonists and antagonists and what are euphemistically called multitarget compounds, that is, drugs which have simultaneous activities on different receptor types (6).

The pharmacokinetics of ergot compounds and the recognition of the so-called first pass effect; drugs released from tightly bound deep compartments, may offer rewarding new approaches to the pharmacotherapy of headache (6).

Calcium Blockers in Vascular Muscle Disorders

The fairly recent appearance of useful calcium entry blockers and their proven efficacy in a number of cardiovascular disorders has suggested that they might also be useful in the therapy of vascular headache, particularly migraine where an initial fall in cerebral blood flow has been demonstrated.

Calcium ions are important in a number of biologic processes and control the rate and the force of contractions of smooth muscle cells. The contractile proteins of these cells depend for activation on the concentration of calcium ions in their cytoplasm. This concentration of ionic calcium depends, in turn, on the entry of calcium ions into the cell. The movement of calcium ions is accomplished through voltage dependent channels, receptor operated channels, sodium/calcium ion exchange systems and ionophore mediated transport systems (8).

One pathogenetic theory currently fashionable suggests that migrainous attacks depend on a sequence of events beginning in the periphery and ending in cerebral vasoconstriction. Platelet aggregation, release of platelet factors, particularly thromboxane A2, focal cerebral vasoconstriction, followed by a reactive vasodilatation associated with headache, is a possible explanation of migraine neglecting, of course, the primary neurogenic aspects of migraine previously emphasized. Calcium channel blockers have antiplatelet aggregation properties and vasodilatory effects, and have been tried as interval therapy in migraine with some success (26). Moreover, anecdotal evidence also suggests that nifedipine sublingually for acute attacks, particularly in patients with a prolonged aura, may also be useful.

But therapeutic measures directed at what is believed by some to be a secondary manifestation of the migrainous diathesis is a priori doomed to partial success. Until the neurogenic origin of vascular headaches is known, the treatment of most patients remains empirical.

Newer Expensive Investigations

Computed tomography (CT) has now become commonplace and affordable. This technique, when first introduced, was used for the study of vascular headache, but few patients showed abnormalities. CT can image cadaver brains, and gives little information about functional changes.

Nuclear magnetic imaging (NMI), positron emission tomography (PET), and brain electrical activity mapping (BEAM) are techniques which give information about function and metabolism. They are now expensive but, like CT, will become affordable in the future and will predictably be applied to the study of headache patients.

REFERENCES

1. Appenzeller, O. (1976): In: The Pathogenesis and Treatment of Headache in Adults and Children, edited by O. Appenzeller, pp. 43-48. Spectrum Publications, Inc., New York.

2. Appenzeller, O. (1984): In: Headache 3/47-, Handbook of Clinical Neurology, edited by F. C. Rose. Elsevier Scientific Publishing Company, Amsterdam.

3. Appenzeller, O., and Atkinson, R. (1983): In: 1st International Headache Congress, Munich, September 1983.

4. Appenzeller, O., Becker, W. J., and Ragaz, A. (1981): Arch. Neurol., 38:302.

5. Appenzeller, O., and Green, R. (1984): In press.

6. Berde, B. (1984): J. Royal Soc. Med., 77:5.

7. Blau, J. N. (1984): J. Neurol. Neurosurg. Psychiat., 47:437.

8. Braunwald, E. (1982): N. Engl. J. Med., 307:1618.

9. Carraway, R., and Leeman, S. E. (1973): J. Biolog. Chem., 248:6854.

10. Epstein, M. T., Hockaday, J. M., and Hockaday, T. D. R. (1975): Lancet, 1:543.

11. Goedert, M. (1984): Trends Neurosci., 7:3.

12. Grant, E. C. G. (1968): Brit. Med. J., 3:402.

13. Hartschuh, W., Weihe, E., and Reinecke, M. (1983): Brit. J. Dermatol., 109:14 (Suppl. 25).

14. Krain, L. S., Levin, J. M., and Shvitz, B. (1978): Cutis, 21:81.

15. Kudrow, L. (1984): Personal communication.

16. Lembeck, F., and Gamse, R. (1982): In: Substance P in the Nervous System, pp. 35-54. Ciba Foundation Symposium 91. Pitman Publ., London.

17. Liberski, P. P., and Prusinski, A. (1982): Headache, 22:115.

18. McIntosh, R. M., Ozawa, T., Persoff, M., and Altshuler, T. H. (1977): N. Engl. J. Med., 296:1265.

19. Ratnoff, O. D. (1980): Seminars in Hematol., 71:192.

20. Rose, D. P., and Braidman, I. P. (1971): Amer. J. Clin. Nutr., 24:673.

21. Russell, M., Dark, K. A., Cummins, R. W., Ellman, G., Callaway, E., and Peeke, H. V. S. (1984): Science, 225:733.

22. Sawyer, M., Kauffman, H., Burnstock, G., and Appenzeller, O. (1984): 5th International Migraine Symposium Proceedings.

23. Severinghaus, J. W., Chiodi, H., Eger, E. I. 2nd, Brandstater, B., and Hornbein, T. F. (1966): Circ. Res., 19:274.

24. Singh, I., Khanna, P. K., Srivastava, M. C., Lal, M., Roy, S. B., and Subramanyam, C. S. V. (1969): N. Engl. J. Med., 280:175.

25. Smith, E. M., and Blalock, J. E. (1981): <u>Proc. Natl. Acad. Sci. (USA)</u>, <u>78</u>:7530.
26. Solomon, G. D., Steel, J. G., and Spaceavento, L. J. (1983): <u>JAMA</u>, <u>250</u>:2500.
27. Somerville, B. W. (1972): <u>Headache</u>, <u>12</u>:93.

Subject Index

Nuclear magnetic resonance (NMR), 34-35

Occipital neuralgia, 5
Opioids, endogenous, 53-54, 141
Oral contraceptives, 70, 72, 73, 83, 90, 172-173
Oxygen, for cluster headache, 123

Paget's disease, 2
Pain perception
  memory for pain, 169-170
  in migraine, 32, 53, 56, 108
  in tension headache, 129
Paracetamol, 76, 97, 98-99
Paresthesia, 9
Pentazocine, 140
Personality, factor in headache
  in children, 154
  cluster headache, 119
  diagnosis, 139-140
  tension headache, 128, 129, 130-131
Phenelzine, 88
Pheochromocytoma, 6
Pizotifen, 84, 97, 101-103, 161
Platelets
  ADP uptake, 26-27
  adenine nucleotide content, 28-29
  aggregation, 26-28, 30, 52, 72, 89
  5-HT uptake, 26-27, 29-30
  migraine and, 26-31, 49, 50-52, 73, 89-90
  in diagnosis, 26, 28, 31
  monamine oxidase, 30-31, 51, 52
  releasing factor, 29-30
Polymyalgia rheumatica, 2
Potassium ions, 58
Pregnancy, 83
Prochlorperazine, 161
Prolactin, 56
Prophylaxis, See also Treatment
  cluster headache, 120-122
  migraine, 54, 55-56, 72-73, 83-90, 97-98, 101-107, 161-162
  tension headache, 133
Propranolol, 72, 85, 86-87, 97, 101, 103-105, 161
Proxibarbal, 90-91
Pseudotumor cerebri, 153
Psychogenic headache, 12, 162, 174

Raeder's paratrigeminal neuralgia, 3
Raphe neurons, 102
Referred pain, 4-5
Reserpine, 88

Sandifer syndrome, 158, 160
Scotomas, in migraine, 9
Serotonin, migraine and, 84
Sex differences
  cluster headache, 12, 116, 118, 124
  migraine, 30-31, 48, 51, 155-157
Shingles, 4
Single photon emission computerized tomography (SPECT), 40
Sinusitis, 5, 153, 170
Sonambulism, 159
Spreading depression, 33, 34, 44-45, 57-58, 60
Status migrainosus, 140-42, 170

See also Migraine
Subarachnoid hemorrage, 6, 143-145
Substance P antagonists, 175
Surgical treatments, for cluster headache, 123-124

Temporal arteritis, 2
Tension headache, See also Muscle contraction headache
  in children, 162
  diagnosis, 12, 82, 131-132
  muscle contraction and, 127-130
  treatment, 87-88, 132-135
Testosterone, cluster headache and, 118
Therapy, See Prophylaxis; Treatment
Thermography, 33
Tic douloureux, 4, 22
Timolol, 103
Tolfenamic acid, 99
Tolosa-Hunt syndrome, 3
Toothache, 169
Tourette's disease, 54
Toxins, headache-causing, 5-6, 23
Trauma, 2, 3, 4, 6, 23, 150-151
  and migraine, 157, 172
Treatment, See also Prophylaxis
  cluster headache, 88-89, 118, 120-124
  emergency-room, 139-147
  migraine
    acupuncture, 135
    drugs, 50, 75-78, 89-91, 97-101, 161
    emergency-room, 140-142
  tension headache, 87-88, 132-135
Triethylperazine, 99
Trigeminal nerve, 3-4
  cluster headache and, 123-124
Tryptophan, 88
Tumors
  in children, 151-153
  diagnosis, 3, 4, 5, 6, 19
Tyramine, and migraine, 30, 83

Urine, in migraine, 49
Urticaria, cerebral, 58

Vasoconstriction
  as migraine cause, See Blood flow
  during migraine treatment, 100-101, 103, 107
Vasodilation, 174-175
  in cluster headache, 117, 118
  as migraine cause, See Blood flow
Verapamil, 103, 106
Vertigo, 159-160
Viloxazine, 87
Visual disorders
  during migraine, 7, 9, 42
  as a consequence of migraine, 69-70
  cause of headache, 4-5, 153

Zimelidine, 86-87

182